FIVE-STAR TRAILS

ASHEVILLE

35 SPECTACULAR HIKES
in the Land of the Sky

JENNIFER PHARR DAVIS

MENASHA RIDGE
PRESS

Five-Star Trails Asheville: 35 Spectacular Hikes in the Land of the Sky
Copyright © 2012, 2018, and 2024 by Jennifer Pharr Davis
All rights reserved
Published by Menasha Ridge Press
Distributed by Publishers Group West
Printed in the United States of America
Third edition, first printing

Cover design by Scott McGrew
Text design by Annie Long
All interior and cover photographs by the author, except on page 196: T. Markley/Shutterstock and
    page 211: chyworks/Shutterstock.com
Cartography and elevation profiles by Steve Jones
Front cover: View toward Craggy Pinnacle (Hike 10, page 65)

Library of Congress Cataloging-in-Publication Data

Names: Davis, Jennifer Pharr, author.
Title: Five-star trails Asheville : 35 spectacular hikes in the land of the sky /
    Jennifer Pharr Davis.
Description: Third edition. | Birmingham, Alabama : Menasha Ridge Press,
    [2024] | Includes index.
Identifiers: LCCN 2023034495 (print) | LCCN 2023034496 (ebook)
    ISBN 9781634043823 (pbk) | ISBN 9781634043830 (ebook)
Subjects: LCSH: Hiking—North Carolina—Asheville Region—Guidebooks. |
    Trails—North Carolina—Asheville Region—Guidebooks. | Asheville Region (N.C.)
    —Guidebooks.
Classification: LCC GV199.42.N662 A754 2023 (print) | LCC GV199.42.N662 (ebook) |
    DDC 796.5109756/88—dc23/eng/20230802
LC record available at https://lccn.loc.gov/2023034495
LC ebook record available at https://lccn.loc.gov/2023034496

 MENASHA RIDGE PRESS
An imprint of AdventureKEEN
2204 First Ave. S., Ste. 102
Birmingham, AL 35233
800-678-7006; fax 877-374-9016

Visit menasharidge.com for a complete listing of our books and for ordering information. Contact us at our
website, at facebook.com/menasharidge, or at twitter.com/menasharidge with questions or comments. To find
out more about who we are and what we're doing, visit blog.menasharidge.com.

SAFETY NOTICE This book is meant only as a guide to select trails in and near Asheville, North Carolina. This
book does not guarantee hiker safety in any way—you hike at your own risk. Neither Menasha Ridge Press nor
Jennifer Pharr Davis is liable for property loss or damage, personal injury, or death that result in any way from
accessing or hiking the trails described in the following pages. Please be especially cautious when walking in
potentially hazardous terrains with, for example, steep inclines or drop-offs. Do not attempt to explore terrain
that may be beyond your abilities. Please read carefully the introduction to this book as well as further safety
information from other sources. Familiarize yourself with current weather reports and maps of the area you
plan to visit (in addition to the maps provided in this guidebook). Be cognizant of park regulations and always
follow them. Do not take chances.

Dedication

To my grandparents, Jones and Polly Pharr. Thank you for sharing your love of the outdoors with me.

And to my husband—always.

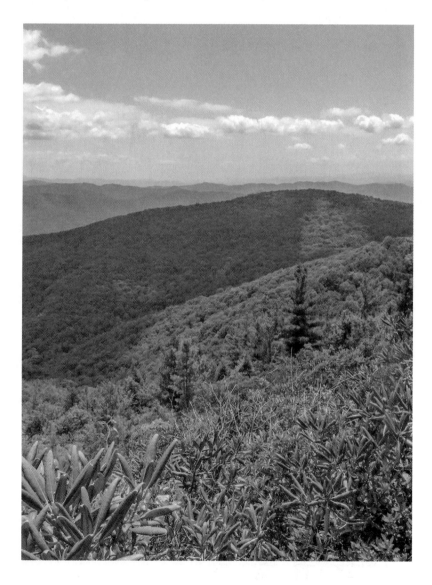

Five-Star Trails: Asheville

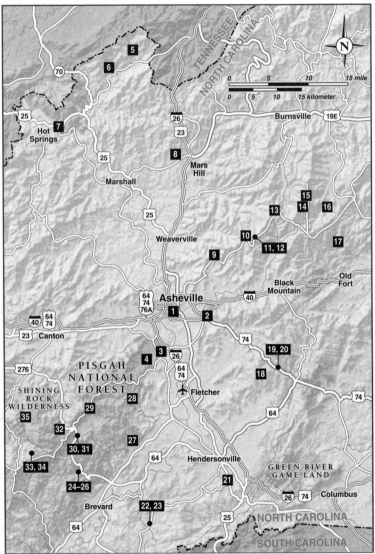

Table of Contents

South   123

West   165

Acknowledgments

THANKS TO MENASHA RIDGE PRESS for producing this third edition of *Five-Star Trails: Asheville*. It struck me while doing work for this guidebook that a lot of credit for the trails in and around Asheville should go to George W. Vanderbilt. The owner of The Biltmore House, he collected, preserved, and managed huge tracts of property as part of his estate and forestry school. Today, those landholdings form a large percentage of Pisgah National Forest, and they also serve as a corridor for the southern portion of the Blue Ridge Parkway.

I want to thank the modern-day agencies that govern those former Vanderbilt holdings, along with the additional public lands and trails in Western North Carolina. Kudos to the private organizations and government bureaus that manage the 2,198-mile Appalachian Trail, the 1,000-mile Mountains-to-Sea Trail, and the 469-mile Blue Ridge Parkway. It is nice to know that your expedition doesn't have to end in Asheville.

Like other outdoors enthusiasts living in the region, I am also indebted to the hardworking employees who manage Pisgah National Forest, Bent Creek Experimental Forest, and the Shining Rock and Middle Prong Wildernesses. However, my biggest thanks goes to the countless volunteers who spend their time maintaining the hundreds of trails that wind through Western North Carolina. I especially appreciate the work of the trail maintainers within the Carolina Mountain Club. Thank you, CMC, for exploring, building, and maintaining the trails near Asheville for more than 80 years!

I also want to personally thank Diamond Brand Outdoors for helping people to get out and explore the wilderness in Western North Carolina and beyond.

And, finally, I want to thank my parents. When I was a young child, they got me started on many of the hikes mentioned in this book. I have many memories of struggling up a mountain slope behind my two older brothers, but I have no doubt that those early adventures gave me a love for the outdoors and the confidence to climb any mountain.

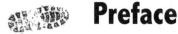 # Preface

WELCOME TO THE THIRD EDITION of this hiking guide to greater Asheville, North Carolina. If you love to hike, there is arguably no better place to enjoy the great outdoors than Asheville. I grew up in these mountains and spent many childhood hours outside with my parents and brothers on local trails. I remember thinking, when I was young, that the "talking" trees at Holmes Educational State Forest really spoke to me; that Mount Pisgah was possibly the tallest, most difficult mountain in the world; and that the coldest water on Earth was found at Sliding Rock.

I never appreciated what a big part of my life these mountains and trails had become until I moved away from the region. Immediately, I began to miss the Southern Appalachians, and soon I realized that these ancient mountains were calling me home. These peaks offer more than just a pretty view or a place to exercise. These mountains are wise overseers who mark the passing of time with delicate springtime buds, the consuming green of summertime, a canopy of fall colors, and a naked vulnerability in winter.

After hiking in many other parts of the United States and on other continents, I often hear people comment that the Southern Appalachians are not as stunning or dramatic as other mountains. I disagree. The highlands around Asheville are some of the oldest and most biodiverse in the world. There may not be a breathtaking mountain vista around every corner, but the intricacies found within the forest shelter can keep a child occupied for hours. It is as if the Appalachians hold their secrets a little closer, revealing them to those who are willing to take the time to explore the terrain.

The challenge of hiking within the Blue Ridge is often much greater than that found in higher mountains. There are more roots, rocks, and texture on the trails near Asheville than on the paths in the proximity of other mountain towns. And despite millions of years of erosion wearing down these surrounding mountains, Western North Carolina can still claim Mount Mitchell, the highest mountain east of the Mississippi River.

The region boasts multiple long-distance trails. They include, of course, the Appalachian Trail—the most famous footpath in the world, and the Mountains-to-Sea Trail. The latter connects the Great Smoky Mountains with the white

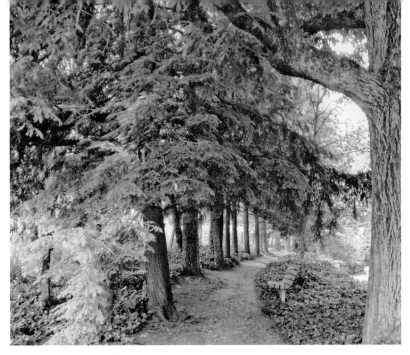

A WELL-DEFINED PATH LEADS FROM THE LAKE TO THE CARL SANDBURG HOME
(Hike 21, page 124).

sand dunes at the eastern end of the state. Near Asheville, the Mountains-to-Sea Trail parallels the ever-popular Blue Ridge Parkway. That national scenic road provides a direct gateway to nature for many of the residents of Asheville and the surrounding areas.

I chose the hikes in this book to showcase the highlights in and around Asheville. I made every attempt to combine the well-known favorites of the region with those less-traveled—but comparably scenic—routes, creating a montage of outdoor experiences for you to indulge in. Although the hiking in this region is not considered easy when compared with the rest of the southeastern United States, the guidebook covers hikes with a wide array of distances, terrains, and difficulties to suit all ages and skill levels. Many of the trail descriptions include suggestions for extending or shortening the prescribed route, providing even more choices.

Still, the most daunting challenge of writing this guidebook was narrowing the hundreds of excursions down to 35 of the *best* day hikes. The Asheville area offers myriad choices that rank high, apropos of the publisher's *Five-Star Trails* series categories (see pages x–xi). As you hike the trails that I've selected, I am sure you will discover more of your own favorites.

Recommended Hikes

Best for Convenience

Best for Geology

Best for History Lovers

Best for Kids

Best for Scenery

Best for Seclusion

Best for Waterfalls

Best for Wildflowers

Best for Wildlife

ONE OF THE REWARDING VIEWS FROM SNOOKS NOSE *(Hike 17, page 102)*

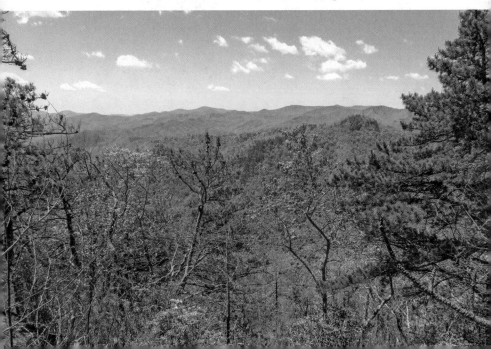

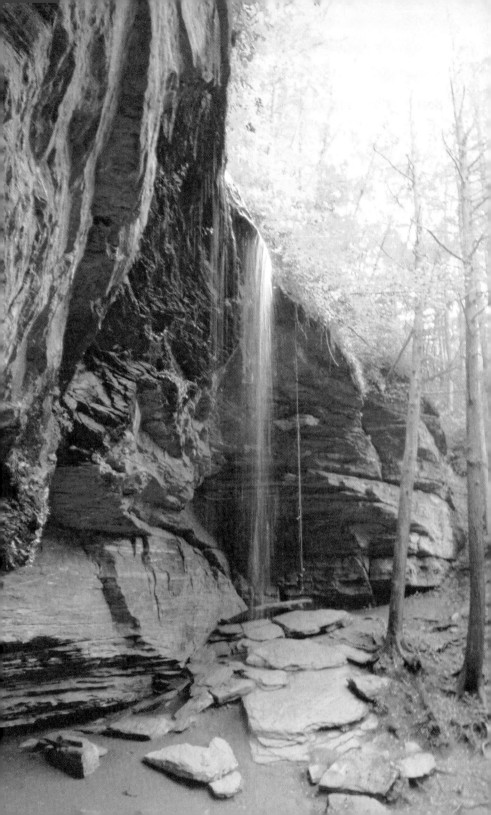

Introduction

About This Book

THE 35 HIKING ROUTES IN *Five-Star Trails: Asheville* are organized with the area's geography in mind. From 5 trails in the central area, the guidebook moves north for 8 trails, east for 5 trails, south for 7 trails, and west for 10 trails. Following is a description of each of these breakouts.

Central

Hooray for so many trails close to the city of Asheville! Numerous folks who work and live in the area make use of these trails on a daily basis, primarily in the Bent Creek Experimental Forest and along Asheville's expanding greenway system. And the forest bordering the city's eastern and western flanks is widely accessible via the Mountains-to-Sea Trail.

North

The Blue Ridge Parkway north of Asheville includes the 6,000-foot peaks along the Craggy Ridgeline and the historic ruins at Rattlesnake Lodge. Most of the hikes in this area take place on or near the Mountains-to-Sea Trail, but a day trip to Hot Springs, North Carolina, will also allow you to take the Appalachian Trail to a gorgeous vista at Lovers Leap, as well as newer Bailey Mountain Preserve. The trek atop Big Firescald Knob delivers another Appalachian Trail experience. Solitude seekers will enjoy remote Hickey Fork.

East

East of Asheville, the hikes in this guidebook typically are not as heavily traveled as their counterparts to the west. Mount Mitchell is an exception, although you can find relative peace and quiet on its trails until you get very close to the summit. Bearwallow Mountain, Florence Nature Preserve, and Wildcat Rock are privately owned hiking destinations open to the public, with views, waterfalls, and biodiversity. Snooks Nose is a very steep, unsung hike with a whopper of a view, while Big Butt Little Butt Hike presents panoramas of the Mount Mitchell

OPPOSITE: **MOORE COVE FALLS EXECUTES ITS CURTAIN DIVE** (*Hike 26, page 149*).

high country. The perky loop hike to Setrock Creek will reward hikers of all ages and abilities.

South

Variety characterizes the routes in this section. Turkey Pen is a multiuse trail-head, hosting equestrians, mountain bikers, and hunters as well as hikers. The trek to Looking Glass Rock is a classic hike to a rewarding vista. Hikers, writers, and families all love to visit Carl Sandburg's Connemara Farms in Flat Rock. And DuPont State Forest offers stunning waterfalls and plenty of trails that are worth exploring time and time again.

West

West of Asheville, this guidebook leads you primarily into Pisgah National Forest, including Shining Rock Wilderness. Here, you will find that the longest and most challenging routes in this guidebook lie west of Asheville, at Shining Rock and Cold Mountain. The west region also features Black Balsam, Sam Knob, and Mount Pisgah—some of the most popular hiking destinations in our area.

How to Use This Guidebook

THE FOLLOWING INFORMATION walks you through this guidebook's organization to make it easy and convenient to plan great hikes.

Overview Map and Regional Maps

The overview map on page iv depicts the location of the primary trailhead for all 35 of the hikes described in this book. The numbers shown on the overview map pair with the table of contents on the facing page. Each hike's number remains with that hike throughout the book. Thus, if you spot an appealing hiking area on the overview map, you can flip through the book and find those hikes easily by their numbers at the top of the first page for each profile. This book is divided into regions, and prefacing each regional chapter is a regional map. These maps provide more detail than the overview map, bringing you closer to the hikes.

Trail Maps and Map Legend

In addition to the overview map, a detailed map of each hike's route appears with its profile. On each of these maps, symbols indicate the trailhead, the complete route, significant features, facilities, and topographic landmarks such

MAP LEGEND

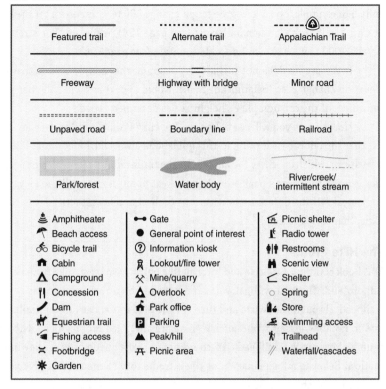

as creeks, overlooks, and peaks. A legend identifying the map symbols used throughout the book appears above.

To produce the highly accurate maps in this book, I used a handheld GPS unit to gather data while hiking each route, and then sent that data to the publisher's expert cartographers.

Despite the high quality of the maps in this guidebook, the publisher and I strongly recommend that you always carry an additional map—or maps— such as the ones noted in each hike profile's "Maps" listing.

Elevation Profiles

This graph represents the rises and falls of the trail as viewed from the side, over the complete mileage of that trail. On the diagram's vertical axis, or height scale, the number of feet indicated between each tick mark lets you visualize the ascent or descent. To avoid making flat hikes look steep and steep hikes appear flat, varying height scales provide an accurate image of each route's hiking difficulty. For example, one hike's scale might change 800 feet, as shown for the hike at Carl Sandburg's Connemara Farms (see page 124), while another stretches nearly 3,000 feet, as shown for Cold Mountain (see page 196).

If the profile does not include the diagram, that simply means that the elevation change is so insignificant that it would appear as a virtually flat path regardless of the cartographer's height scales described above.

However, as you will see below, in "The Hike Profile" section, the key-info list that introduces each route in this guidebook always includes a text line for "elevation," which specifies the altitude at the trailhead. This item also notes the elevation at the route's peak—or at the lowest point, if the trailhead elevation *is* the peak. (If the difference between the highest and lowest altitudes is negligible, that also is stated.)

The Hike Profile

This book contains a concise and informative narrative of each hike from beginning to end. The text will get you from a well-known road or highway to the trailhead, through the twists and turns of the hike route, back to the trailhead, and to notable nearby attractions, if there are any. Each profile opens with the route's star ratings, Trailhead GPS coordinates, and a lineup of other key information. Below is an explanation of the introductory elements that give you a snapshot of each of the 35 routes in *Five-Star Trails: Asheville.*

STAR RATINGS

As with all of Menasha Ridge Press' regional hiking guidebooks, authors for the *Five-Star Trails* series are locally based, experienced outdoors writers. As part of their research, they personally hike a variety of trails—often creating unique routes by marrying sections of different trails.

To determine worthy selections for this series, authors assess the qualities of each route in the five categories shown at right. Each trail must average high ratings among the five categories; or it must be outstanding in one or more of these categories. For example, the author may award a trail only one star for "Condition" but five stars for "Scenery" and include it in the book. Why? Because, based on the author's own trek, it is well worth hiking the "rocky, overgrown, or often muddy" path in order to witness and savor its "unique, picturesque panorama."

Following is the explanation for the rating system of one to five stars in each of the five categories.

FOR SCENERY:

★ ★ ★ ★ ★	Unique, picturesque panoramas
★ ★ ★ ★	Diverse vistas
★ ★ ★	Pleasant views
★ ★	Unchanging landscape
★	Not selected for scenery

FOR TRAIL CONDITION:

★ ★ ★ ★ ★	Consistently well maintained
★ ★ ★ ★	Stable, with no surprises
★ ★ ★	Average terrain to negotiate
★ ★	Inconsistent, with good and poor areas
★	Rocky, overgrown, or often muddy

FOR CHILDREN:

★ ★ ★ ★ ★	Babes in strollers are welcome
★ ★ ★ ★	Fun for anyone past the toddler stage
★ ★ ★	Good for young hikers with proven stamina
★ ★	Not enjoyable for children
★	Not advisable for children

FOR DIFFICULTY:

★ ★ ★ ★ ★	Grueling
★ ★ ★ ★	Strenuous
★ ★ ★	Moderate (won't exhaust you, but you'll know you've been hiking)
★ ★	Easy, with patches of moderate
★	Good for a relaxing stroll

FOR SOLITUDE:

★ ★ ★ ★ ★	Positively tranquil
★ ★ ★ ★	Spurts of isolation
★ ★ ★	Moderately secluded
★ ★	Crowded on weekends and holidays
★	Steady stream of individuals and/or groups

TRAILHEAD GPS COORDINATES

As noted in "Trail Maps" (see pages 2–3), I transmitted data from a handheld GPS unit to the publisher's cartographers. In addition to its use in creating this book's maps, that information verified the GPS coordinates—the inter-section of the lines of latitude (north) and longitude (west)—to place you at the trailhead.

In some cases, you can drive to a parking point within viewing distance of that trailhead. Other hikes require a short walk to reach the trailhead from a parking area. Either way, the trailhead coordinates are given from the point where you will begin hiking.

Pertinent to visualizing the GPS coordinates, the latitude and longitude grid system is likely quite familiar to you, but here is a refresher:

Imaginary lines of latitude—called parallels and approximately 69 miles apart from each other—run horizontally around the globe. Each parallel is indicated by degrees from the equator (established to be 0°): up to 90°N at the North Pole and down to 90°S at the South Pole.

Imaginary lines of longitude—called meridians—run perpendicular to latitude lines. Longitude lines are likewise indicated by degrees: starting from 0° at the Prime Meridian in Greenwich, England, they continue to the east and west until they meet 180° later at the International Date Line in the Pacific Ocean. At the equator, longitude lines are approximately 69 miles apart, but that distance narrows as the meridians converge toward the North and South Poles.

GPS coordinates may be expressed in a variety of formats. This book uses decimal degrees, the format used by Google Maps.

As an example, see the GPS coordinates for Hike 1, the French Broad River Greenway: 35.569719, -82.564931. The first number represents the lati-tude at which the trailhead is located, and the second number represents the longitude. Simply plug these values into your GPS device to navigate directly to the trailhead.

For more on GPS technology, visit usgs.gov.

DISTANCE & CONFIGURATION

The distance shown is for the complete hike, round-trip. (Unless otherwise specified, the mileage does not include any options to shorten or extend the hike, but these are addressed in the hike description.)

Configuration defines the trail as a loop, an out-and-back, a figure eight, or a balloon.

HIKING TIME

Unlike distance, which is measured, hiking time is an estimate. Every hiker has a different pace. In this guidebook, the hiking time is based on a pace of about 1.75–2 miles per hour. There are some adjustments for steepness, rough terrain, and high elevation. And there is some time built in for a quick breather here and there, but any prolonged break (such as lunch or swimming) will add to the hike time. Also keep in mind seasonal daylight hours, so that you don't find yourself hiking back to the trailhead in the dark, and remember that forested canopies greatly block the fading daylight.

HIGHLIGHTS

Waterfalls, historic sites, or other features that draw hikers to the trail are listed here.

ELEVATION

Unless the route is virtually flat—in which case only one elevation will be listed—two elevation points are always indicated: one for the trailhead and another for the highest or lowest altitude on that route. For most hikes, you will ascend from the trailhead, but in some cases, the trailhead is the route's peak, and you descend from there. (Also see "Elevation Profiles" on page 3.)

ACCESS

Fees or permits required to hike the trail and trail-access hours are indicated here.

MAPS

This item recommends sources in addition to the maps in this guidebook, and hikers are strongly urged to consult these references.

FACILITIES

This section alerts you to restrooms, phones, water, picnic tables, and other basics at or near the trailhead.

WHEELCHAIR ACCESS

For each hike, you will readily see whether or not it is accessible for wheelchair users.

COMMENTS

Assorted nuggets of information, such as whether or not dogs are allowed on the trails, appear here.

CONTACTS

Phone numbers and websites listed here are handy for checking trail conditions and gleaning other day-to-day information.

OVERVIEW, ROUTE DETAILS, NEARBY ATTRACTIONS, AND DIRECTIONS

Each profile contains a complete narrative of the hike: "Overview" gives you a quick summary of what to expect on that trip. The "Route Details" section guides you on the hike, start to finish. In "Nearby Attractions," you will learn of area sites that you might like, such as restaurants, museums, or other trails. "Directions" will get you to the trailhead from a well-known road or highway.

Weather

HIKING IS A GREAT ACTIVITY to enjoy in Asheville throughout the year.

Hiking the trails around Asheville in autumn should be on everyone's to-do list. The forest lights up like a fireworks show, and blueberries and blackberries grow along or near most paths. Animal sightings are also prevalent during this season, as many of the animals are trying to eat as much as possible before the long, cold winter.

Springtime is a favorite season for many hikers, as wildflowers and wildlife begin to appear around the trail. Mid-May, mountain laurels and flaming azaleas accent many trails with beautiful pink and orange blooms.

During summer, highland trails are a great place to escape the heat. Waterfall hikes become especially desirable during this season. However, mountain vistas are sometimes less spectacular, as a summer haze can obscure the distant peaks.

In winter, road access by car to the trailheads for many of the best hikes in the region becomes difficult or impossible if the Blue Ridge Parkway closes. Note that real-time road openings and closures can be accessed through the

MONTHLY WEATHER AVERAGES FOR ASHEVILLE, NORTH CAROLINA							
MONTH	HI TEMP	LO TEMP	RAIN	MONTH	HI TEMP	LO TEMP	RAIN
JAN	46°F	27°F	3.07"	JUL	84°F	64°F	2.97"
FEB	50°F	29°F	3.19"	AUG	83°F	62°F	3.34"
MAR	58°F	36°F	3.89"	SEP	77°F	56°F	3.01"
APR	67°F	44°F	3.16"	OCT	68°F	45°F	2.40"
MAY	74°F	52°F	3.53"	NOV	58°F	37°F	2.93"
JUN	81°F	60°F	3.24"	DEC	50°F	30°F	2.59"

parkway's website, nps.gov/blri. Check "Alerts in Effect" near the top of the homepage. But several of these trails are still reachable if you are willing to drive to them on winding back roads or to hike in on approach trails. The bare trees of December, January, and February provide incredible views that are not available the rest of the year.

Water

HOW MUCH IS ENOUGH? Well, one simple physiological fact should convince you to err on the side of excess when deciding how much water to pack: you can sweat nearly 2 quarts of fluid each hour you walk in the heat, more if you hike uphill in direct sunlight and during the hottest time of the day. A good rule of thumb is to hydrate prior to your hike, carry (and drink) 16 ounces of water for every mile you plan to hike, and hydrate again after the hike. For most people, the pleasures of hiking make carrying water a relatively minor price to pay to remain safe and healthy. So pack more water than you anticipate needing, even for short hikes.

If you are tempted to drink "found water," do so with extreme caution, whether it is a stream or lake. *Giardia* parasites contaminate many water sources and cause the dreaded intestinal giardiasis that can last for weeks after ingestion. For information, visit the Centers for Disease Control website at cdc.gov /parasites/giardia.

In any case, effective treatment is essential before using any water source found along the trail. Boiling water for 2–3 minutes is always a safe measure for camping, but day hikers can consider iodine tablets, approved chemical mixes, filtration units rated for *Giardia*, and UV filtration. Some of these methods (e.g., filtration with an added carbon filter) remove bad tastes typical in stagnant water, while others add their own taste. Carry a means of purification to help in a pinch or if you realize you have underestimated your consumption needs.

Clothing

WEATHER, UNEXPECTED TRAIL CONDITIONS, fatigue, extended hiking duration, and wrong turns can individually or collectively turn a great outing into a very uncomfortable one at best—and a life-threatening one at worst. Thus, proper attire plays a key role in staying comfortable and, sometimes, in staying alive. Here are some helpful guidelines:

★ Choose silk, wool, or synthetics for maximum comfort in all of your hiking attire—from hats to socks and in-between. Cotton is fine if the weather remains dry and stable, but you won't be happy if it gets wet.

★ Always wear a hat, or at least tuck one into your day pack or hitch it to your belt. Hats offer all-weather sun and wind protection as well as warmth if it turns cold.

★ Be ready to layer up or down as the day progresses and the mercury rises or falls. Today's outdoor wear makes layering easy, with such designs as jackets that convert to vests and zip-off or button-up legs.

★ Wear hiking boots or sturdy hiking sandals with toe protection. Flip-flopping on a paved path in an urban botanical garden is one thing, but never hike a trail in open sandals or casual sneakers. Your bones and arches need support, and your skin and nails need protection.

★ Pair that footwear with quality socks! If you prefer not to sheathe your feet when wearing hiking sandals, tuck the socks into your day pack; you may need them if the weather plummets or if you hit rocky turf and pebbles begin to irritate your feet. And, in an emergency, if you have lost your gloves, you can adapt the socks into mittens.

★ Don't leave rainwear behind, even if the day dawns clear and sunny. Tuck into your day pack, or tie around your waist, a jacket that is breathable and either water-resistant or waterproof. Investigate different choices at your local outdoor retailer. If you are a frequent hiker, ideally, you'll have more than one rainwear weight, material, and style in your closet to protect you in all seasons in your regional climate and hiking microclimates.

Essential Gear

TODAY, YOU CAN BUY outdoor vests that have up to 20 pockets shaped and sized to carry everything from toothpicks to binoculars, or, if you don't aspire to feel like a burro, you can neatly stow all of these items in your day pack or backpack. The following list showcases never-hike-without-them items—in alphabetical order, for easy reference:

★ Duct tape: One of those small rolls you get at the drugstore will do. It can hold gear together if needed, and it's good for preventing blisters if you apply it to the hot spot early enough.

★ Extra clothes: Bring raingear, a warm hat, gloves, and a change of socks and shirt.

★ Extra food: Pack trail mix, granola bars, or other high-energy foods.

★ Flashlight or headlamp: Include an extra bulb and batteries.

★ Insect repellent: For some areas and seasons, this is extremely vital.

★ *Maps and high-quality compass:* Even if you know the terrain from previous hikes, don't leave home without these tools, and consult and carry more than one map (in addition to those in this guidebook). Though phones have GPS receivers in them, lack of service can render the GPS-based maps inoperable.

★ *Matches (ideally, wind- and waterproof) and/or a lighter:* A fire starter is also a good idea.

★ *Pocketknife and/or a multitool:* Never hike without one of these implements.

★ *Sunscreen:* Note the expiration date on the tube or bottle.

★ *Water:* As emphasized more than once in this book, bring more than you think you will drink; depending on your destination, you may want to bring a water bottle and filter for purifying water in the wilderness in case you run out.

★ *Whistle:* This little gadget is more effective than your voice in an emergency.

First Aid Kit

IN ADDITION TO THE ITEMS ABOVE, those below may appear overwhelming for a day hike. But any paramedic will tell you that the products listed here, in alphabetical order, are just the basics. The reality of hiking is that you can be out for a week of backpacking and acquire only a mosquito bite—or you can hike for an hour, slip, and suffer a bleeding abrasion or broken bone. Fortunately, these items will collapse into a very small space, and convenient, prepackaged kits are available at your pharmacy and online.

Consider your intended terrain and the number of hikers in your party before you exclude any article cited below. A botanical garden stroll may not inspire you to carry a complete kit, but anything beyond that warrants precaution. When hiking alone, you should always be prepared for a medical need. And if you are a twosome or with a group, one or more people in your party should be equipped with first aid material.

★ Ace bandages or other joint wraps

★ Adhesive bandages (such as Band-Aids)

★ Antibiotic ointment (Neosporin or the generic equivalent)

★ Athletic tape

★ Benadryl or the generic equivalent, diphenhydramine (in case of allergic reactions)

★ Blister kit (such as Moleskin/Spenco Second Skin)

★ Butterfly-closure bandages

★ Epinephrine in a prefilled syringe (for people known to have severe allergic reactions to such things as bee stings; usually by prescription only)

★ Gauze (one roll and a half dozen 4x4-inch pads)

★ Hydrogen peroxide or iodine

★ Ibuprofen or acetaminophen

General Safety

THE FOLLOWING TIPS may have the familiar ring of your mother's voice as you take note of them:

★ *Always let someone know where you will be hiking* and how long you expect to be gone. It's a good idea to give that person a copy of your route, particularly if you are headed into any isolated area. Let them know when you return.

★ *Always sign in and out of any trail registers provided.* Don't hesitate to comment on the trail condition if space is provided; that's your opportunity to alert others to any problems you encounter.

★ *Never exclusively count on a smartphone for your safety.* Reception may be spotty or nonexistent on the trail, especially in deep valleys enveloped by mountains, a common occurrence around Asheville.

★ *Always carry food and water,* even for a short hike. And bring more water than you think you will need. (I cannot say that often enough!)

★ *Stay on designated trails.* Even on the most clearly marked trails, there is usually a point where you have to stop and consider which direction to head. If you become disoriented, don't panic. As soon as you think you may be off track, stop, assess your current direction, and then retrace your steps to the point where you went astray. Using a map, a compass, GPS, and this book, and keeping in mind what you have passed thus far, reorient yourself, and trust your judgment on which way to continue. If you become absolutely unsure of how to continue, return to your vehicle the way you came in. Should you become completely lost and have no idea how to return to the trailhead, remaining in place along the trail and waiting for help is most often the best option for adults and always the best option for children.

★ *Always carry a whistle.* It may be a lifesaver (or at least a major stress-reducer) if you do become lost or sustain an injury.

★ *Be especially careful when crossing streams.* Whether you are fording the stream or crossing on a log, make every step count. If you have any doubt about maintaining your balance on a log, ford the stream instead: use a trekking pole or stout stick for balance and face upstream as you cross. If a stream seems too deep to ford, turn back. Whatever is on the other side is not worth risking your life. By the way, trekking poles improve balance on the trail as well as when crossing streams.

★ *Be careful at overlooks.* While these areas may provide spectacular views, they are potentially hazardous. Stay back from the edge of outcrops and be absolutely sure of your footing; a misstep can mean a nasty and possibly fatal fall.

★ *Look up!* Standing dead trees and storm-damaged living trees pose a real hazard to hikers. These trees may have loose or broken limbs that could fall at any time. Be mindful of this when walking beneath trees, and when choosing a spot to rest or enjoy your snack.

★ *Know hypothermia symptoms.* Shivering and forgetfulness are the two most common indicators of this stealthy killer. Hypothermia can occur at any elevation, even during summer, especially when the hiker is wearing lightweight cotton clothing. If symptoms present themselves, get to shelter, hot liquids, and dry clothes ASAP.

★ *Ask questions.* National and state forest and park employees are there to help. It's a lot easier to ask advice beforehand, and it will help you avoid a mishap away from civilization when it's too late to amend an error.

★ *Most important of all, take along your brain.* A cool, calculating mind is the single-most important asset on the trail. Think before you act. Watch your step. Plan ahead. Avoiding accidents before they happen is the best way to ensure a rewarding and relaxing hike.

Watchwords for Flora and Fauna

FOLLOWING IS SOME SPECIFIC ADVICE about dealing with the various hazards that come with wandering through the ecosystem. They are listed in alphabetical order.

BLACK BEARS In primitive and remote areas, assume bears are present; in more developed sites, check on the current bear situation prior to hiking. Most encounters are food related, as bears have an exceptional sense of smell and not particularly discriminating tastes. While this is of greater concern to backpackers and campers, on a day hike, you may plan a lunchtime picnic or just munch on an energy bar or other snack from time to time. So remain aware and alert.

Though attacks by black bears are rare indeed, the sight or approach of a bear will give anyone a start. If you encounter a bear while hiking, remain calm and never turn your back to run away. Instead, make loud noises to scare off the bear and back away slowly.

MOSQUITOES Insect repellent and/or repellent-impregnated clothing are the only simple methods available to ward off these pests. In some areas, mosquitoes are known to carry the West Nile virus, so all due caution should be taken to avoid their bites.

POISON IVY, OAK, AND SUMAC   Recognizing and avoiding poison ivy, oak, and sumac is the most effective way to prevent the painful, itchy rashes associated with these plants. Poison ivy occurs as a vine or groundcover, three leaflets to a leaf; poison oak occurs as either a vine or shrub, also with three leaflets; and poison sumac flourishes in swampland, each leaf having 7–13 leaflets. Urushiol, the oil in the sap of these plants, is responsible for the rash. Within 14 hours of exposure, raised lines and/or blisters will appear on the affected area, accompanied by a terrible itch. Refrain from scratching because bacteria under your fingernails can cause an infection. Wash and dry the affected area thoroughly, applying a calamine lotion to help dry out the rash. If itching or blistering is severe, seek medical attention. If you do come into contact with one of these plants, remember that oil-contaminated clothes, hiking gear, or pets can easily cause an irritating rash on you or someone else, so wash not only any exposed parts of your body but also clothes, gear, and pets, if applicable.

SNAKES   Rattlesnakes, cottonmouths, copperheads, and coral snakes are among the most common venomous snakes in the United States, and hibernation season is typically October into April. In the Asheville hiking area, you will possibly encounter rattlesnakes, cottonmouths, and copperheads. However, the snakes you most likely will see while hiking will be nonvenomous species and subspecies. The best rule is to leave all snakes alone, give them a wide berth, and make sure any hiking companions (including dogs) do the same.

For the best protection when hiking, stick to well-used trails and wear over-the-ankle boots and loose-fitting long pants. Rattlesnakes like to bask in the sun and won't bite unless threatened. Do not step or put your hands where you cannot see, and avoid wandering around in the dark. Step onto logs and rocks, never over them, and be especially careful when climbing rocks. Always avoid walking through dense brush or willow thickets.

TICKS   Ticks often live in areas around brush and tall grass, where they seem to be waiting to hitch a ride on a warm-blooded passerby. Adult ticks are most active April into May and again October into November. Among the varieties of ticks, the black-legged tick, commonly called the deer tick, is the primary carrier of Lyme disease. Wear light-colored clothing, so ticks can be spotted before they make it to the skin. And be sure to visually check your hair, back of neck, armpits, and socks at the end of the hike. During your post-hike shower, take a moment to do a more complete body check. For ticks that are already embedded, removal with tweezers is best. Use disinfectant solution on the wound.

Hunting

SEPARATE RULES, REGULATIONS, AND LICENSES govern the various hunting types and related seasons. Though there are generally no problems, hikers may wish to forgo their trips during the big-game seasons, when the woods suddenly seem filled with orange and camouflage. Before hiking, check the website of the area's managing body to see if hunting season is in effect, especially during late autumn.

Regulations

TRAIL REGULATIONS IN THE ASHEVILLE REGION are dependent on the governing body of each specific hiking path. However, here are some general guidelines:

★ *Unless specific signs or instructions at the trailhead indicate otherwise,* hikers should assume that dogs have to remain on leashes of less than 6 feet in length. Many hikers are uncomfortable with other people's dogs off-leash, and it is not fair to ruin their hikes because your pooch wants to run free—whether or not leashes are required. Small children are especially vulnerable to unleashed dogs tearing down the trail.

★ *If there is a trailhead information kiosk,* be sure to check the board for pertinent information or recent trail reroutes.

★ *If there is a trail register,* as noted in "General Safety" (see page 12), be sure to sign in and leave your pertinent information before starting the hike.

Trail Etiquette

ALWAYS TREAT THE TRAIL, WILDLIFE, AND FELLOW HIKERS WITH RESPECT. Here are some reminders.

★ *Plan ahead in order to be self-sufficient at all times.* That means carrying necessary supplies for changes in weather or other conditions. A well-executed trip is a satisfaction to you and to others.

★ *Hike on open trails only.*

★ *Respect trail and road closures* (ask if not sure), avoid possible trespassing on private land, and obtain all permits and authorization as required. Also, leave gates as you find them or as marked.

★ *Be courteous to other hikers, bikers, equestrians, and others* you encounter on the trails.

★ *Never spook animals.* An unannounced approach, a sudden movement, or a loud noise startles most animals. A surprised animal can be dangerous to you, to others, and to itself. Give them plenty of space.

★ Observe the YIELD signs that are displayed around the region's trailheads and back-country. They advise hikers to yield to horses, and bikers to yield to both horses and hikers. A common courtesy on hills is that hikers and bikers yield to any uphill traffic. When encountering mounted riders or horse packers, hikers can courteously step off the trail, on the downhill side if possible. Speak to the riders before they reach you and do not dart behind trees. You are less spooky if the horse can see and hear you. Resist the urge to pet horses unless you are invited to do so.

★ Stay on the existing trail and do not blaze any new trails.

★ Be sure to pack out what you pack in, whether you are on a day hike with just a tis-sue and a small lunch sack or on a longer trek with a backpack full of supplies. No one likes to see the trash someone else has left behind. Just think what a difference it would make if everyone picked up just one piece of trash each time they hit the trail.

★ To emphasize: ALWAYS practice Leave No Trace principles. Visit lnt.org for more information. Try to leave the trail in the same condition as you found it—or better.

Tips for Enjoying Hiking in the Asheville Area

THE BEST WAY TO ENJOY YOUR HIKE is to come to the trailhead prepared. And take your time to enjoy the spectacular trails of the Asheville area and its surroundings.

If you are hiking in a group, do not try to keep up with the fastest hiker. Instead, allow each person to go at their own speed. Hike your own hike, as the saying goes. Or, if you wish to stay together, make sure that the pace is comfort-able for everyone.

Another way to enjoy the hike is to make sure that you are properly fueled before starting the trip. If you are hungry or thirsty at the outset of your trek, then it is unlikely you will have much energy or much fun on the trail.

Also, remember that the temperature in Asheville is often much warmer than on top of the surrounding mountaintops. On your hike, be prepared for a 10–20 degree drop in temperature and stronger winds than are present on the valley floor.

If you are a fan of spotting wildlife, consider planning your trek for the hours that coincide with dawn and dusk. This is the best time to spot bears, turkey, and deer. Pay particular attention to the trail during the heat of the day, as this is the time when snakes typically enjoy stretching across the trail and sunbathing.

OPPOSITE: **PROPER GEAR EASES THE DIFFICULTY OF ACCESSING VIEWS LIKE THIS ONE AT SHINING ROCK WILDERNESS** *(Hike 35, page 196).*

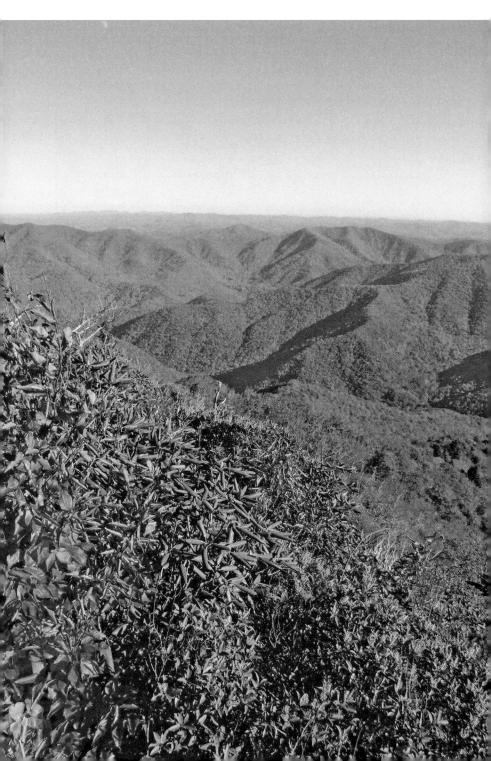

Central

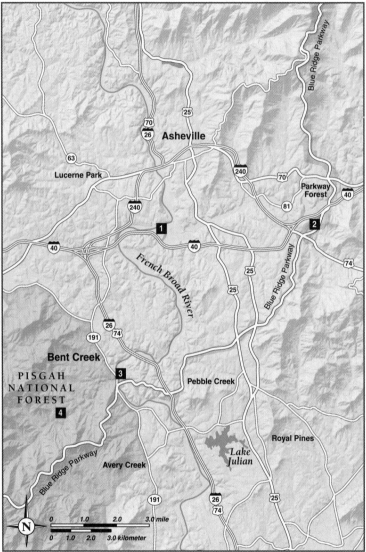

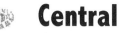 # Central

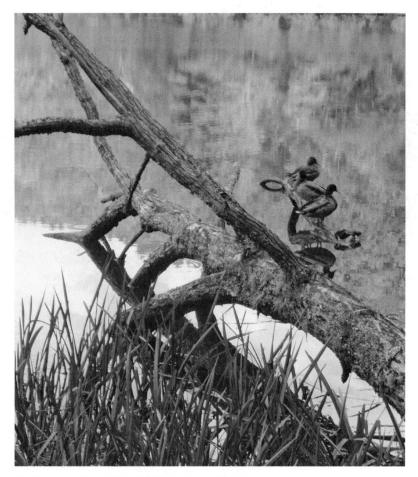

DUCKS REST ON A FALLEN TREE AT LAKE POWHATAN *(Hike 4, see page 33).*

French Broad River Greenway

SCENERY: ★ ★ ★
TRAIL CONDITION: ★ ★ ★ ★ ★
CHILDREN: ★ ★ ★ ★ ★
DIFFICULTY: ★ ★
SOLITUDE: ★

JOGGERS, WALKERS, AND HIKERS LIKE US ENJOY THE FRENCH BROAD RIVER GREENWAY.

TRAILHEAD GPS COORDINATES: 35.569719, -82.564931

DISTANCE & CONFIGURATION: 2.9-mile balloon loop

HIKING TIME: 1.7 hours

HIGHLIGHTS: Four parks, French Broad River views, people-watching

ELEVATION: Around 1,980 feet throughout trek

ACCESS: No fees or permits required

MAPS: French Broad River Greenway West; USGS *Asheville*

FACILITIES: Restrooms, picnic tables, benches at trailhead and other points of hike

WHEELCHAIR ACCESS: Yes, entire route

CONTACTS: City of Asheville Transportation Department, 828-259-5805, ashevillenc.gov/department /transportation/greenways

Overview

Enjoy this fine urban trek in the heart of Asheville, where the French Broad River Greenway links four city parks. Start with a warm-up circuit at big and busy French Broad River Park, then make your way to Amboy Riverfront Park to pass through newer Karen Cragnolin Park before reaching Carrier Park, where you loop your way back to the trailhead. Additional segments of greenway on either end make extending this wheelchair-accessible adventure a breeze.

Route Details

Sometimes life gets in the way of doing wilderness hikes among the far-flung mountains around Asheville. When this happens to me, rather than shirking the trail altogether, I gather up the family (if possible) and head to one of Asheville's expanding networks of greenways. The French Broad River Greenway is a good choice, as it travels along the river and links several parks together. The starting point, French Broad River Park, is often full of fellow parkgoers and great for people-watching. Of course, upon arriving, you will be one of the people being watched!

A kiosk will help orient you to the park, the French Broad River, and the greenways all about. Facing the river, you will head left (north) just past where the French Broad River has made a big bend after accepting the waters of the Swannanoa River. Trees shade the asphalt path. All manner of activity happens here, from fishing to frolicking, from picnicking to yoga, from in-line skating to reading. You will soon come near the enclosed dog park. Talk about frolicking! You next come to the river and will turn south at a connector, linking to the north portion of the French Broad River Greenway West. The roiling, fun-to-paddle French Broad is to your left, and the French Broad River Greenway East runs along the far bank. Asheville is just chock-full of urban greenways.

Your hike soon passes under Amboy Road, then turns west with the curve of the water to enter Amboy Riverfront Park. Enjoy close-up river views before reaching a paddle launch and alternative parking area at 0.8 mile. You soon leave Amboy Riverfront Park to reach 5-acre Karen Cragnolin Park. Why so many parks next to one another? The answer is the parks were developed at different times, each one coming into existence independently. Karen Cragnolin Park opened in 2023 and was named after the local advocate for such things as riverside parks and greenways. Note that the riverside seating at this preserve was formerly a junkyard. After the property purchase in 2006, it took years of remediation to get the land into shape to become a park. Over 100,000 tons of concrete were removed from the site, as well as smashed cars, etc.!

French Broad River Greenway

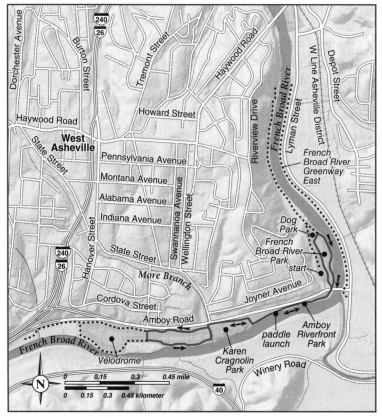

The greenway twists through Karen Cragnolin Park amid a mix of meadows and trees; at 1.1 miles the trail bridges Moore Branch near where it flows into the French Broad. This waterway's drainage, West Asheville, is in an entirely urban area, contributing its flow for better or worse into the French Broad. Then you are in Carrier Park, with multiple developed facilities, highlighted by a Velodrome, where bicyclers circle and circle a banked track, testing their speed. The French Broad River Greenway continues a westerly flat course, linking to spur nature trails. At 1.4 miles, you come to the Michigan Avenue entrance to the park, with a large parking area. This is a good place to begin looping back toward French Broad River Park, though you could easily continue on the French Broad River West Greenway to Hominy Creek River Park or simply loop back at the far end of Carrier Park.

From the Michigan Avenue park entrance, turn toward the river and join the riverside trail winding east. Pass the park pavilion. Rejoice in aquatic panoramas as you wind in and out of shade. At 1.8 miles, return to Karen Cragnolin Park. From this point you will be backtracking toward French Broad River Park. After walking back under Amboy Road, split left toward the trailhead, completing the urban hike at 2.9 miles and proving that Asheville's greenways can provide a quick getaway when you just don't have time for a major hike.

Nearby Attractions

It is a short walk or drive from the trailhead to the heart of Asheville's River Arts District, where artists aplenty are located with open studios, ready for your visit. For more information, visit riverartsdistrict.com.

Directions

From Exit 2, US 19 Business/US 23 Business, on I-240/I-26 in Asheville, join Haywood Road eastbound to turn right (south) on Hanover Street and follow it 0.4 mile to turn left on State Street. Follow State Street for 0.7 mile to turn left on Amboy Road. Drive 0.5 mile, then make a quick left turn onto Riverview Drive, then a quick right turn into French Broad River Park.

Destination Center Track Trail

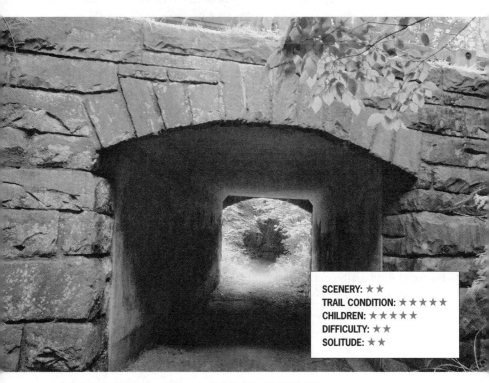

SCENERY: ★ ★
TRAIL CONDITION: ★ ★ ★ ★ ★
CHILDREN: ★ ★ ★ ★ ★
DIFFICULTY: ★ ★
SOLITUDE: ★ ★

THE TRAIL TRAVELS UNDERNEATH THE BLUE RIDGE PARKWAY.

TRAILHEAD GPS COORDINATES: 35.565667, -82.486550

DISTANCE & CONFIGURATION: 1.4-mile loop

HIKING TIME: 1 hour

HIGHLIGHTS: The Blue Ridge Parkway Destination Center

ELEVATION: 2,264' at the trailhead, 2,121' south of the parkway

ACCESS: Free and always open, but vehicle access to this hike is unavailable when the Blue Ridge Parkway is closed. Check nps.gov/blri for real-time road closures.

MAPS: Blue Ridge Parkway Milepost 384 TRACK Trail; USGS *Oteen*

FACILITIES: Restrooms; water; visitor center with displays, videos, exhibits, and general Information

WHEELCHAIR ACCESS: Yes, at the Destination Center

COMMENTS: The Destination Center is open daily, 9 a.m.–5 p.m.; closed Thanksgiving, Christmas, and New Year's Days.

CONTACTS: 828-348-3400, nps.gov/blri

Overview

This hike is especially well suited for those with children—like me—and for those who are children at heart. Start at the Destination Center to learn about the Blue Ridge Parkway through educational exhibits and interactive technology. When it is time to move on to the trailhead, you will see a child-friendly sign that describes the hike and provides information and activity brochures that correspond with the ensuing 1.4-mile loop.

Route Details

The state-of-the-art, LEED-certified Destination Center offers an enjoyable beginning to this hike. Kids and adults will lose track of time among the visually appealing exhibits and interactive games. One highlight is the large, sliding LED screen that allows you to virtually travel the length of the Blue Ridge Parkway.

After exploring the family-oriented Destination Center, walk to the opposite side of the parking lot to the Track Trail. There you will find an attractive sign mounted on a stone arch. Pamphlets available beneath the sign are designed to help younger hikers identify plants and insects along the trail.

The Track Trail and informational brochures are part of an initiative called Kids in Parks. The Blue Ridge Parkway Foundation created the program. The mission statement of the Kids in Parks program as stated on kidsinparks .com is "engaging kids and families in outdoor recreation to foster lifelong wellness and meaningful connections to public lands."

As part of the initiative, the Blue Ridge Parkway Foundation has constructed or designated several Track Trails near the Blue Ridge Parkway and beyond, which provide children with interactive and educational materials to help them make the most of their hikes. In addition to the trailhead information and brochures, your child can log on to kidsinparks.com to participate in the online Track Trail program. The following hike at the Blue Ridge Parkway Destination Center was the first Track Trail created (back in 2009) and serves as a pilot for similar trails along the Blue Ridge Parkway. Track Trails have expanded to 12 states.

From the Track Trail sign, travel into the woods on a dirt path behind the trailhead marker. In a few feet, the trail will split. Begin the loop by turning right and continuing slightly downhill. After 0.1 mile the blazes that mark the

Destination Center Track Trail

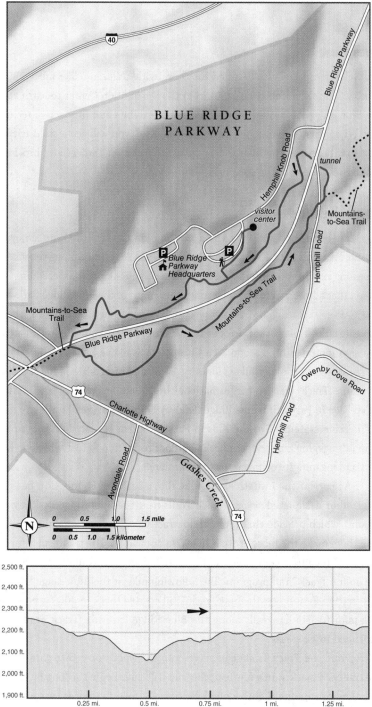

trail will lead past a large gray building to the right. This structure serves as the main headquarters for the Blue Ridge Parkway and its rangers, landscape architects, and park superintendent; they work to preserve and protect the National Scenic Road, which extends 469 miles from the Great Smoky Mountains near Cherokee, North Carolina to Rock Fish Gap near Waynesboro, Virginia.

After 0.5 mile you will exit the woods at the Blue Ridge Parkway, and the trail continues on the opposite side of the road. If you are hiking with children, exercise extra caution before crossing, as commuter cars often zip down the parkway. Across the road, the Track Trail joins the white-blazed Mountains-to-Sea Trail (MST) and veers east. The next 0.5-mile stretch is great for children to search for bugs such as granddaddy longlegs or grasshoppers. It is also a good area for using the brochures to help identify the different types of ferns that line the path, including hay-scented fern, bracken fern, and Christmas fern.

On this part of the path, 1 mile from the trailhead, you will come to a junction. The MST continues uphill to the right, but you will want to go straight and rejoin the blazes that lead back toward the Destination Center. The correct path will lead you through a tunnel underneath the parkway. The hiker tunnel is popular with photographers on social media. In winter this tunnel often has bedazzling icicles adorning the front and back entrances.

Back on the other side of the parkway, you will pass a gravel ATV trail on your right that leads directly to the Destination Center. Your group may be eager to revisit the Destination Center, but to complete the loop you will veer left and follow the trail another 0.2 mile. Then turn right on the short trail stem that leads back to the Destination Center parking lot.

Directions

From downtown Asheville, take I-240 east toward Oteen. From I-240, turn left onto Exit 9 toward I-40 and the Blue Ridge Parkway, then immediately veer left onto US 74A. After 0.5 mile turn right onto the Blue Ridge Parkway. Travel the parkway north 0.5 mile and then turn left onto Hemphill Knob Road. Park at the Destination Center.

Rocky Cove

SCENERY: ★ ★ ★
TRAIL CONDITION: ★ ★ ★ ★ ★
CHILDREN: ★ ★ ★
DIFFICULTY: ★ ★ ★ ★
SOLITUDE: ★ ★ ★

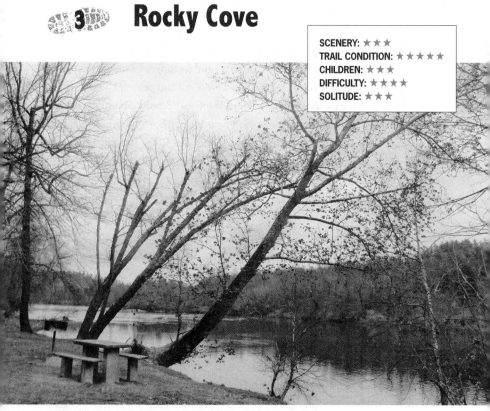

THE WEST BANK OF THE FRENCH BROAD RIVER

TRAILHEAD GPS COORDINATES: 35.501456, -82.593147

DISTANCE & CONFIGURATION: 5.5-mile loop

HIKING TIME: 3 hours

HIGHLIGHTS: The historic Shut-In Trail and the well-groomed and scenic paths within the
North Carolina Arboretum

ELEVATION: 2,000' at trailhead, 2,564' at Hardtimes Road

ACCESS: Bent Creek Experimental Forest is free and always open. The North Carolina Arboretum is open April–
October, 8 a.m.–9 p.m.; November–March, 8 a.m.–7 p.m.; there is a parking fee that varies by vehicle type.

MAPS: National Geographic #780 *Pisgah Ranger District;* USGS *Bent Creek, Skyland*

FACILITIES: Portable toilet at the parking lot next to the arboretum entrance

WHEELCHAIR ACCESS: Yes, at several buildings on the arboretum property,
including the Visitor Education Center

COMMENTS: Although the arboretum charges a parking fee, it generously allows hikers to access the property
on foot free of charge. This hike starts outside the arboretum and does not require a hiker to pay, but visitors
will want to consider purchasing a yearly membership to fully enjoy the arboretum facilities and programs.

CONTACTS: North Carolina Arboretum, 828-665-2492, ncarboretum.org

Overview

Starting at the French Broad River, this hike follows a steep ascent on the historic Shut-In Trail, which George Vanderbilt used to access his Buck Spring hunting lodge near Mount Pisgah. After 2 miles the trail intersects Hardtimes Road and then follows the Rocky Cove drainage down into the scenic and well-maintained North Carolina Arboretum. Once inside the arboretum, the trail parallels Bent Creek and passes beside the National Native Azalea boundary before leaving the arboretum boundary to conclude the hike at the French Broad River.

Route Details

Start this hike at Bent Creek River and Picnic Park off of NC 191, very near the Blue Ridge Parkway on-ramp and North Carolina Arboretum entrance. Parking area picnic tables provide a nice spot to view the river or enjoy a bite to eat before or after the hike.

To begin the loop, walk to the north end of the parking lot, where Bent Creek empties into the French Broad River. Look upstream and locate the blazed trail leading underneath NC 191 and beside Bent Creek. Follow this path for a short distance to its end point at the Blue Ridge Parkway on-ramp. Carefully cross the road at a southwest angle to locate the Shut-In Trail. The Shut-In Trail coincides with the white-blazed Mountains-to-Sea Trail.

This portion of the Shut-In Trail marks the very beginning of George W. Vanderbilt's route up the ridgeline to his hunting cabin near Mount Pisgah. (Other portions of the 16-mile Shut-In Trail can be explored on the Mount Pisgah via Buck Spring Lodge hike; see page 166.) The route starts on a relatively level trail to the North Carolina Arboretum boundary. Once the fences that mark the arboretum property line come into view, veer south and uphill on a sharp switchback. The switchback will lead through an unlocked gate that marks the Bent Creek Experimental Forest boundary.

Upon entering Bent Creek, you will be greeted with an uphill route that parallels the Blue Ridge Parkway but travels far enough above the road to avoid most of the noise from motorized vehicles (loud motorcycles are the exception to this rule). The forest comprises primarily tall oak, maple, and poplar trees. There is very little underbrush. In winter, when the leaves are off the trees, views of South Asheville and the French Broad River extend below.

Rocky Cove

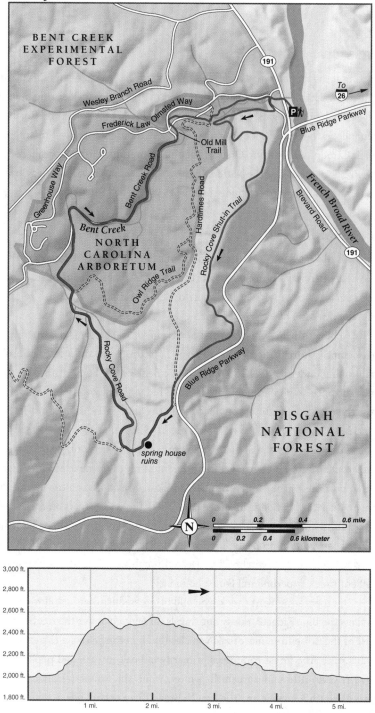

After straining your calf muscles for 0.5 mile, it will come as a welcome relief when the trail begins to level out on the ridge. At 1.6 miles the trail intersects an old roadbed and continues to the left. From there, you will skirt the east side of now-wooded Glenn Bald before connecting with Hardtimes Road. This is a main artery leading through neighboring Bent Creek, but on this hike you will only follow Hardtimes Road for a brief 0.3 mile. After hiking past a spring and the ruins of a rock reservoir on your left, you will leave Hardtimes Road and veer north to descend on Rocky Cove Road.

Rocky Cove Road, although not quite as well maintained as Hardtimes Road, is yet another wide dirt road that is closed to vehicular traffic. The next 1 mile of walking will follow Rocky Cove Road along the western drainage basin of the Shut-In Ridge. The road passes through several acres of white pine trees—part of the forestry and logging experimentation at Bent Creek. A few minutes later, you will reach a gate that separates the experimental forest from the North Carolina Arboretum.

Pass through the gate and veer left to continue on Rocky Cove Road, as the Owl Ridge Trail enters on your right. At 3.8 miles Rocky Cove Road terminates. Turn right on Bent Creek Road. Bent Creek Road stays near the meandering banks of Bent Creek and parallels Bent Creek Trail. If you prefer singletrack to wide dirt roads, then consider hiking Bent Creek Trail. Both the trail and road will lead to the National Native Azalea Repository at 4.3 miles. Observe the native shrubs, which usually bloom in late spring and early summer, before continuing northeast on Bent Creek Road.

At the next intersection, leave Bent Creek Road and turn right onto Old Mill Trail. The path will take you over Bent Creek and then under the arboretum main drive before arriving at a dirt road and arboretum parking lot. Turn left to access the parking area and travel to the northwest corner of the lot to continue the hike on a maintained but unmarked footpath.

The trail now stays between Bent Creek and the arboretum entrance for 0.2 mile, until it reaches a small waterway that intersects Bent Creek from the north. At this point, cross over the guardrail and walk along the arboretum entrance for 0.1 mile to reach the Blue Ridge Parkway on-ramp. Immediately on the other side of the on-ramp, a blazed spur trail will lead underneath NC 191 and back to the trailhead at the Bent Creek River and Picnic Park.

Directions

From downtown Asheville, travel I-26 south to Exit 33. Turn right off the exit onto NC 191. Travel 2.1 miles on NC 191. Immediately after passing the North Carolina Arboretum and Blue Ridge Parkway on-ramp to your right, turn left into the Bent Creek River and Picnic Park.

From South Asheville, take the Blue Ridge Parkway to mile marker 393 and exit right toward the North Carolina Arboretum. At the end of the on-ramp, turn right. The Bent Creek River and Picnic Park will be on your left.

LOOKING OUT ON THE FRENCH BROAD RIVER

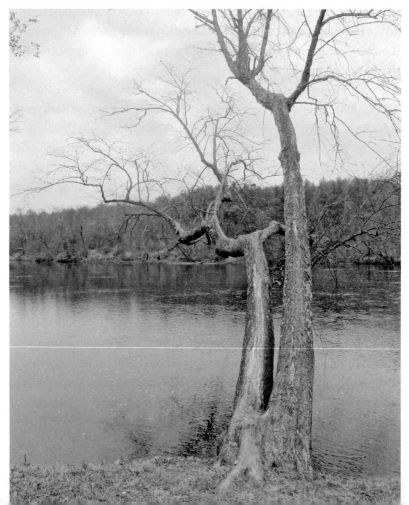

Lake Powhatan

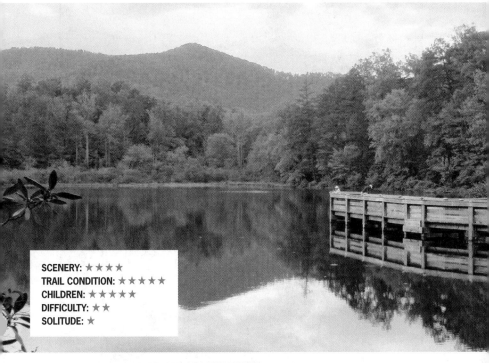

SCENERY: ★ ★ ★ ★
TRAIL CONDITION: ★ ★ ★ ★ ★
CHILDREN: ★ ★ ★ ★ ★
DIFFICULTY: ★ ★
SOLITUDE: ★

A VIEW OF LAKE POWHATAN AND THE FISHING PIER

TRAILHEAD GPS COORDINATES: 35.487836, -82.624255

DISTANCE & CONFIGURATION: 1.6-mile balloon

HIKING TIME: 1 hour

HIGHLIGHTS: Views of Lake Powhatan, the fishing pier, and seasonal swim area

ELEVATION: 2,163' at the trailhead, 2,168' at Lake Powhatan

ACCESS: The trails at Bent Creek Experimental Forest are free and always open. Lake Powhatan Recreation Area is open 8 a.m.–sunset and requires an auto entry fee. (The following hike avoids this fee by entering the boundary on foot.)

MAPS: National Geographic #780 *Pisgah Ranger District*; USGS *Skyland, Dunsmore Mountain*

FACILITIES: Pit toilets at the trailhead; portable toilets at the fishing pier

WHEELCHAIR ACCESS: Yes, at the fishing pier, via Lake Powhatan Recreation Area

COMMENTS: The beach at Lake Powhatan is open for swimming 10 a.m.–8 p.m. Memorial Day through Labor Day, when the lifeguard is on duty.

CONTACTS: Bent Creek Experimental Forest, srs.fs.usda.gov/bentcreek; Lake Powhatan Recreation Area, fs.usda.gov/nfsnc

Lake Powhatan

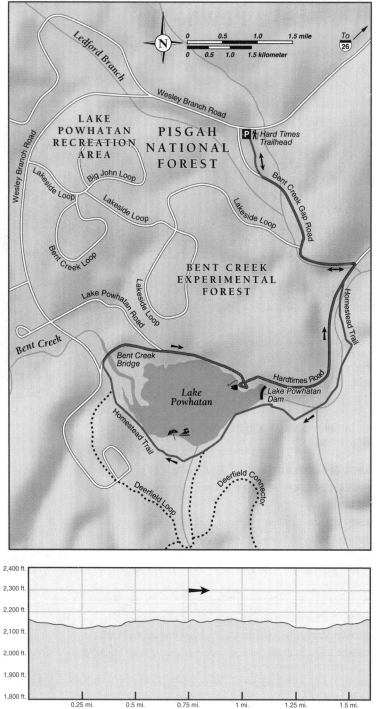

Overview

The level terrain and varied scenery on this trail make it ideal for families with young children. Starting at the Hardtimes Trailhead, the route follows both gravel roads and a singletrack trail to the dam at Lake Powhatan. From the dam, the path leads through a rhododendron tunnel to the beach on the north end of the lake, and then to the fishing pier on the opposite shore. Then the route travels on a forest road through towering hardwood trees back to the parking area.

Route Details

This hike takes you through Bent Creek Experimental Forest and Lake Powhatan Recreation Area. By parking and beginning the hike at the Hardtimes Trailhead in Bent Creek Experimental Forest, you will avoid a parking fee in the Lake Powhatan Recreation Area. However, if you wish to access the recreation area directly, or if there are individuals in your party who want to see the lake but are unable to hike, then it is possible to pay the vehicle entry fee and drive directly to Lake Powhatan and the wheelchair-accessible fishing pier.

To begin your hike, walk south from the Hardtimes Trailhead and away from Wesley Branch Road. You will pass a U.S. Forest Service gate that is typically closed. Continue on the gravel road past the gate. You are now hiking on Bent Creek Gap Road, a gravel treadway that is closed to vehicular traffic, except for authorized vehicles. However, it is a popular road for mountain bikers, so don't be surprised if one comes whizzing behind you. Peculiarly, even off-road unicyclists train in Bent Creek. Talk about having good balance!

After passing the Hardtimes Connector dirt trail on your right, you will come to an intersection with another wide gravel road. Bent Creek Gap Road continues to the left, but you want to turn right to access Hardtimes Road. Once on Hardtimes Road, you will follow Bent Creek for a few hundred feet and then turn left and cross the creek on a cement bridge. On the other side of the bridge, take an immediate right to leave the gravel road and join the orange-blazed Homestead Trail.

The Homestead Trail will continue to parallel Bent Creek until you reach the dam at Lake Powhatan. Falling water sounds indicate your proximity to the dam. There is an unmarked spur trail leading a few feet to the left that reveals great views of the dam and Lake Powhatan.

Leaving the dam, continue on the Homestead Trail and contour the banks of Lake Powhatan. Even though you are traveling very close to the water, the lake may not be visible through the dense rhododendron and mountain laurel thicket lining the path, especially when these evergreens are in bloom in spring and early summer.

After hiking 0.8 mile, arrive at a trail junction. The trail to the left leads to Deerfield Loop, but you want to veer right and continue on the Homestead Trail. A few hundred feet past the trail junction, leave the forest behind and enter an open field at the west end of the lake. From there, the recreation area's swim beach stands out. If you are hiking in the summer, the beach is a great place to take a quick dip before moving on down the trail. However, even in the off-season, the sandy shoreline provides an alluring resting spot to enjoy a snack and observe some of the resident ducks that make Lake Powhatan their home.

When you are ready to resume hiking, continue along the banks of the lake and locate the blazes leading back into the forest on the north end of the beach. Ahead, pass the other end of Deerfield Loop. Soon join a short, wooded walk near the lake and then reach a large wooden bridge spanning Bent Creek and the surrounding wetlands. Walk across the bridge and stay extra vigilant as you peer into the wetlands to your left. Scan for signs of beaver activity. In recent years otters have been spotted in this area.

On the opposite side of the bridge, a short connector trail leads past a utility shed to join a gravel road. Turn right on the gravel road and follow it to the fishing pier on the east end of the lake. The pier is open for fishing from the first Saturday in April to the last day in February. The lake is hatchery-supported and stocked with trout, but in order to test your luck with a fishing pole, you will need a state fishing license. Even without a license, it is fun to watch other anglers reel in their latest catch.

After leaving the lake, continue east on the gravel road, along the north bank of Bent Creek. At the same time that you depart the fishing pier parking area and reenter the forest you will also reenter Bent Creek Experimental Forest. At this point, the gravel road you are hiking transitions to the start of Hardtimes Road. Follow this road back past the cement bridge over Bent Creek, and then take your next left onto Bent Creek Gap Road. This road will lead you on a 0.3-mile slight ascent back to the Hardtimes Trailhead and parking area.

Nearby Attractions

Lake Powhatan Recreation Area offers reservable overnight camping and day-time recreational opportunities, with modest fees for day use or overnight camping. Facilities include flush toilets, showers, and picnic tables.

Directions

From I-26 take Exit 33 and turn left onto NC 191/Brevard Road. Travel 1.9 miles and then turn right onto Bent Creek Ranch Road. In 0.2 mile the road makes a sharp left turn and becomes Wesley Branch Road. Follow Wesley Branch Road 2 miles; the Hardtimes Trailhead will be on your left.

THE LAKE POWHATAN DAM CREATES AN ARTIFICIAL WATERFALL.

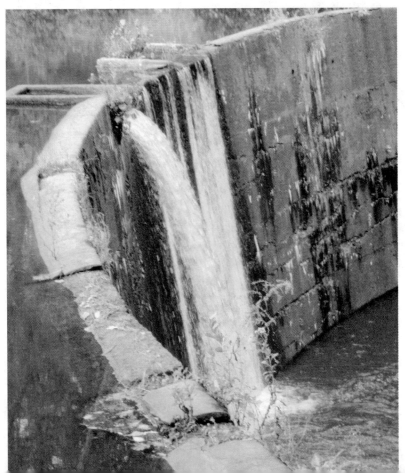

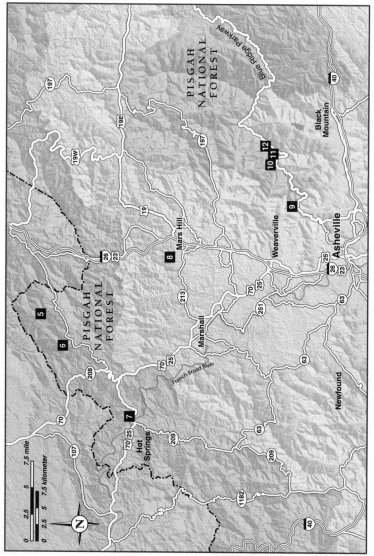

North

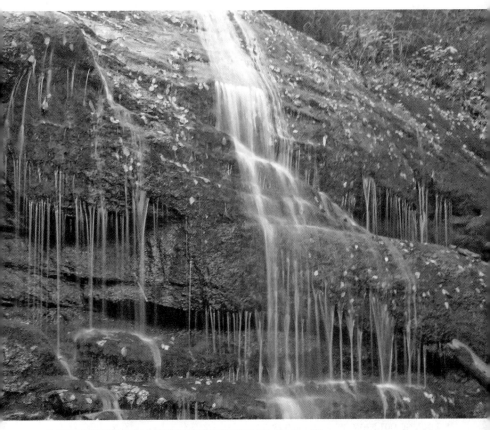

HICKEY FORK FALLS IS A SELDOM-SEEN SPILLER *(Hike 6, page 45).*

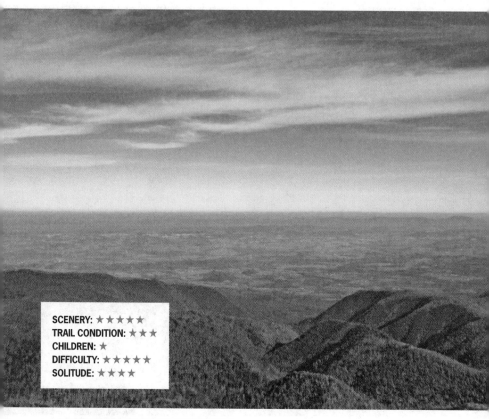

SCENERY: ★ ★ ★ ★ ★
TRAIL CONDITION: ★ ★ ★
CHILDREN: ★
DIFFICULTY: ★ ★ ★ ★ ★
SOLITUDE: ★ ★ ★ ★

LOOKING OUT FROM BIG FIRESCALD KNOB

TRAILHEAD GPS COORDINATES: 36.023434, -82.652887

DISTANCE & CONFIGURATION: 10.2-mile loop

HIKING TIME: 6.5–7.5 hours

HIGHLIGHTS: Cascade, 360-degree rocky views

ELEVATION: 2,400' at trailhead, 4,530' at highest point

ACCESS: No fees or permits required

MAPS: National Geographic #782 *French Broad and Nolichucky Rivers (Cherokee and Pisgah National Forests);* USGS *Greystone*

FACILITIES: None

WHEELCHAIR ACCESS: None

CONTACTS: Pisgah National Forest; Appalachian Ranger District, 828-689-9694, fs.usda.gov/nfsnc

Overview

This loop takes place in the Shelton Laurel Backcountry of the Pisgah National Forest. The Jerry Miller Trail takes you to a 100-foot waterslide before opening onto Whiteoak Flats, a closing meadow. Ascend to the Appalachian Trail (AT). Walk the stony knife-edge delineating North Carolina and Tennessee. Incredible 360-degree views unveil atop Big Firescald Knob, a half mile of continuous outcrops opening into the Tar Heel State and the Volunteer State. A steep trip down Fork Ridge takes you back to the trailhead.

Route Details

Note the trailhead memorial to Jerry Miller, a Carolinian and advocate of national forests. Bridge Big Creek on the Jerry Miller Trail, heading downstream. This flat will fill with wildflowers in spring. Scale a ridge dividing Big Creek from Whiteoak Flats Branch, avoiding an old route that crosses private property. Look for white trilliums here by the score. Turn into Whiteoak Flats Branch watershed at 0.3 mile. Head up the steep-sided valley among rhododendrons, sourwoods, pines, and magnolias.

The valley of Whiteoak Flats Branch closes in at 0.9 mile. Keep an eye out for a noteworthy cascade to your left. Here, a long slide pours down the hollow, then drops in stages before slowing. Winter's barren trees reveal the full 100-foot fall. The valley shuts, and you take a short log bridge over now-gentle Whiteoak Flats Branch at 1.2 miles. Hop a tributary at 1.3 miles, then open onto what remains of Whiteoak Flats meadow. The former homestead is growing over with briers, pines, and tulip trees, yet the surrounding ridges are still visible.

Whiteoak Flats meadow ends at 1.6 miles, and you'll open onto a second, smaller clearing at 1.7 miles. Stay with the blazed trail, careful to avoid old roadbeds spurring from the primary trail. Take a sharp left at 2.1 miles. An old road goes straight here. The proper path is blazed with paint; old roads fade and/or become overgrown. Rise to a dry ridge with black gum, pine, and mountain laurel. The Jerry Miller Trail then turns into upper Chimney Creek valley shaded by rhododendron arbors.

Tributaries of upper Chimney Creek sporadically spill over the trail. Rise to grassy Huckleberry Gap and a four-way intersection at 4 miles. To your right is a short path to a campsite. To your left, a signed trail leads atop a knob, then

Big Firescald Knob

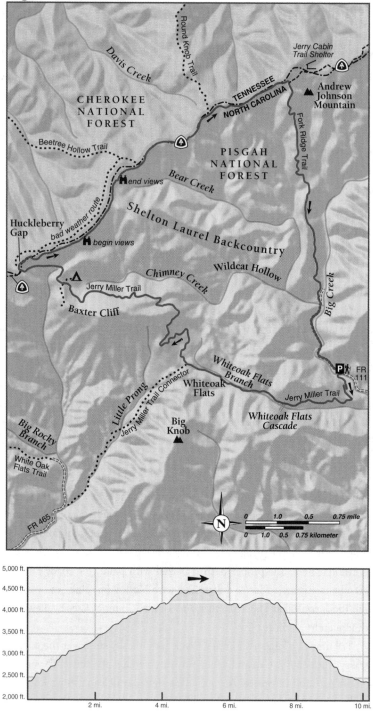

sharply down to Baxter Cliff after 0.4 mile, with a view of Whiterock Cliff and Hickey Fork below.

The Jerry Miller Trail leaves straight from Huckleberry Gap, curving around upper Hickey Fork to reach the AT at 4.5 miles. Turn right, northbound on the AT, to quickly find another intersection. Here, the old AT, now dubbed Bad Weather Route, stays left, while you stay right on the Exposed Ridge Route, the newer AT section. Begin ascending among pale stone bluffs, boulders, and steps shaded by beech and yellow birch. Make a stony switchback at 4.7 miles and head along the state line crest among wind-stunted hardwoods.

At 5.1 miles, rise to Big Firescald Knob and begin a remarkable half mile of hiking. A jagged, irregular rock backbone rises above the trees. Looking into Tennessee, steep mountainsides give way to a patchwork quilt of farms and fields. Looking into North Carolina, ridge after ridge extends easterly. During winter, look for the Jerry Miller Trail climbing toward Huckleberry Gap below, under the leafless trees. Stone steps, a result of backbreaking trail construction, lead through the craggy crest. Diminutive windswept trees find a home in rock fissures, as do undersized rhododendrons, blueberries, mountain laurels, and greenbriers. The going is slow, but maybe that is as it should be, given the incredible splendor. The AT enters more woods than rock at 5.6 miles.

Open to a rock slab and a north view of Big Butt and Green Ridge Knob, then find another overlook of Greene County, Tennessee, at 5.7 miles. Dip to meet the Bad Weather Route at 6 miles. The rocky tread relents to tall woods and an undulating track. This area traverses the Bald Mountains, named for cattle-grazed meadows that once adorned its crests. Today, the forest has regenerated, and an amazing number of painted trilliums and trout lilies carpet the forest floor in April.

At 6.7 miles a road-like trail leads left to Round Knob picnic area. Drift into a gap at 7.2 miles, then circle around the right side of Andrew Johnson Mountain. At 7.4 miles reach the Fork Ridge Trail (if you go too far, you will reach the Jerry Cabin trail shelter after 0.25 mile). Turn right onto Fork Ridge Trail and begin a steep descent. Drop over 1,000 feet in the next mile, flanked by rhododendrons. Make a couple of upticks along the way, emerging in a trailhead parking area on Forest Road 111 at 9.4 miles. From here, follow the forest road along trout-filled, sparkling Big Creek, crossing Chimney Creek by road ford at 9.5 miles, then Big Creek at 9.8 miles. Reach the Jerry Miller trailhead at 10.2 miles, finishing the circuit.

Nearby Attractions

The Shelton Laurel Backcountry has other trails that link to each other and the AT for multiple loop possibilities.

Directions

From Asheville, take I-26 north to Exit 19A/Marshall. Then follow US 25/US 70 for 21 miles. Turn right onto NC 208 West and follow it 3.4 miles. Turn right on NC 212 East and follow it 10.9 miles. Look for the Carmen Church of God and turn left onto Big Creek Road. Follow Big Creek Road for 1.2 miles. The road seems to end near a barn. Here, angle left onto FR 111, taking the gravel road over a small creek, passable by most passenger cars at normal flows. Enter the national forest. At 0.4 mile beyond the barn, turn left onto a spur to dead-end at the signed Jerry Miller trailhead.

SCANNING INTO TENNESSEE FROM THE OPEN CRAGS OF BIG FIRESCALD KNOB

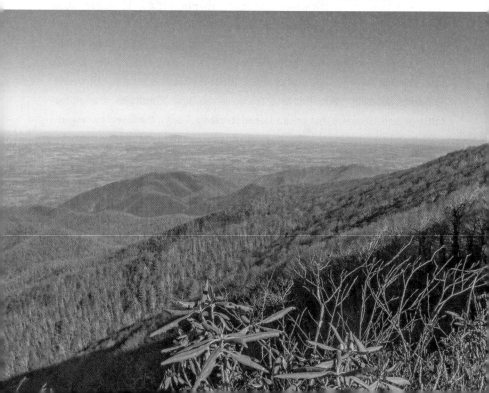

6

Hickey Fork Loop

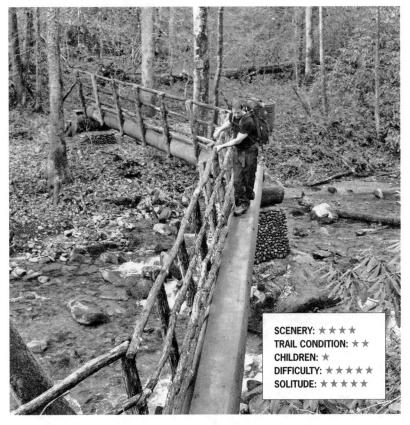

SCENERY: ★ ★ ★ ★
TRAIL CONDITION: ★ ★
CHILDREN: ★
DIFFICULTY: ★ ★ ★ ★ ★
SOLITUDE: ★ ★ ★ ★ ★

CROSSING THE BRIDGE OVER EAST PRONG HICKEY FORK

TRAILHEAD GPS COORDINATES: 35.994533, -82.704617

DISTANCE & CONFIGURATION: 7-mile loop

HIKING TIME: 4–5 hours

HIGHLIGHTS: Waterfalls, solitude

ELEVATION: 2,220' at trailhead, 4,060' at highest point

ACCESS: No fees or permits required

MAPS: National Geographic #782 *French Broad and Nolichucky Rivers (Cherokee and Pisgah National Forests);* USGS *White Rock, Greystone*

FACILITIES: None

WHEELCHAIR ACCESS: None

CONTACTS: Pisgah National Forest, Appalachian Ranger District, 828-689-9694, fs.usda.gov/nfsnc

Hickey Fork Loop

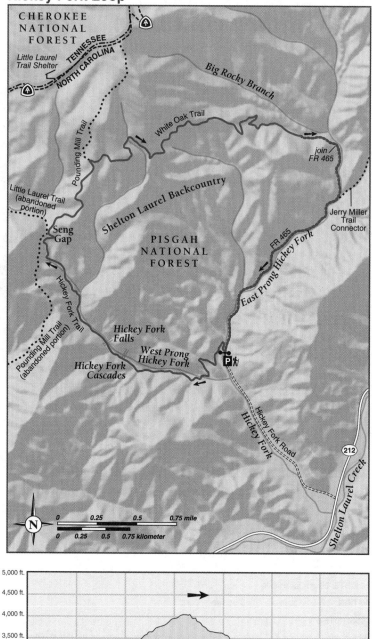

Overview

Solitude lovers will enjoy this stimulating circuit. Set in the Shelton Laurel Backcountry of the Pisgah National Forest, this hike takes you on lesser-used trails through the Hickey Fork watershed. First, ascend West Prong Hickey Fork, passing two significant waterfalls, as well as many lesser cascades, before rising to Seng Gap. Continue toward the North Carolina–Tennessee crest before breaking off and descending toward East Prong Hickey Fork. Reach a remote forest road and make an easy walk back to the trailhead. Winter views add to the trek.

Route Details

This is one of those hikes that makes me ask, "Why don't Ashevillians hike this more often?" The loop has scenic waterfalls and solitude, and it will test hikers due to its lesser-used state, which means a sometimes-faint trailbed, trailside brush, and sporadic blown-down trees. However, the physical beauty more than makes up for the imperfect character of the trail.

Walk up Forest Road 465, passing around a metal gate. Just ahead, the Hickey Fork Trail leaves left, immediately spanning East Prong Hickey Fork on a log bridge with handrails. After crossing East Prong, the slender path heads upstream through rhododendrons before turning away from the creek at 0.1 mile. Work around a low ridge, then join a tributary of West Prong Hickey Fork. This now-old reroute keeps the trail on national forest property. Reach and rock-hop West Prong Hickey Fork at 0.5 mile.

Head upstream on a slender singletrack in lush forest under which lie doghobble, ferns, and an ocean of rhododendrons. Trickling branches cross over the trail, adding volume to West Prong Hickey Fork. Ascend the narrowing valley and come to your first visible fall—Hickey Fork Cascades—at 1.1 miles. This long, sloping cataract flows over a smooth rock bed, dropping in excess of 100 feet. Be careful here. A slide down this wild waterfall would not end well.

Above, the stream falls in pools and drops. Come to a classic curtain-type cataract at 1.3 miles—Hickey Fork Falls. It starts sloped but then dives over a wide rock ledge, crashing during its 35-foot descent. The fact that there is but a scant path to the base of this impressive pour-over testifies to the underuse of this trail. These are remarkable, name-worthy waterfalls! At 1.7 miles the trail leaves West Prong Hickey Fork to the left, ascending a tributary. Gain 400 feet in a very steep 0.3 mile and then open onto a cove, leaving the evergreen thickets behind.

Circle around the upland cove, which is filled with tulip and magnolia trees, and then arrive at level Seng Gap at 2.3 miles. Pay attention here. To your left, the abandoned portion of the Pounding Mill Trail leaves for Pounding Mill Creek. Straight ahead, the abandoned Little Laurel Trail heads for Little Laurel Creek. Our hike leaves right, following an old roadbed, joining the still-maintained portion of the Pounding Mill Trail. Angle upward, northeasterly, to find another saddle at 2.6 miles. Keep rising to a signed trail junction at 2.9 miles. Here, Hickey Fork Trail heads left about a mile for the AT and the state line, while our hike turns right, joining another old roadbed on the White Oak Trail. Cruise easterly. In winter, enjoy views of Round Mountain, just above Seng Gap, and other nearby knobs and distant mountains.

Turn into a hollow, and, at 3.3 miles, the White Oak Trail abruptly leaves right from the old roadbed. Descend to cross a tributary of Hickey Fork at 3.4 miles. This is an interesting area. Here, the very wide branch trickles through

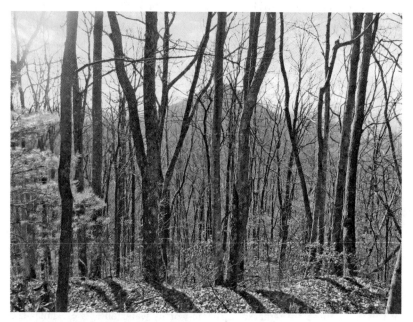

GAZING EAST FROM THE WHITE OAK TRAIL

a boulder field. Use the rocks to dryfoot it across the flow, then turn downstream on a narrow path, as the water crashes below. At 3.6 miles the White Oak Trail makes an abrupt left and begins a long, slow, foot-friendly descent on the south-facing slope of Seng Ridge, cloaked in pines, oaks, and mountain laurel. As you leave Seng Ridge, catch views of the Baxter Cliffs (in winter).

At 4.4 miles the White Oak Trail comes to a closed logging road. Don't go for the wide logging road. Instead, make a sharp left into the valley of Big Rocky Branch, still on singletrack, curving gently to reach the wider lower valley. Keep downhill, breaking out onto FR 465 at 5 miles. Here, FR 465 dead-ends to your left. You keep straight, descending FR 465, with clear East Prong Hickey Fork putting on an aquatic show, powered by gravity. The little-traveled and often-closed road makes for easy hiking. At 5.8 miles an old road bridge on the left crosses bouldery East Prong Hickey Fork and is now an unofficial connector to the Jerry Miller Trail.

This hike keeps downstream on FR 465, bridging East Prong at 6.7 miles. You are now on the east bank. At 7 miles reach the forest road gate and the end of this solitude-filled hike.

Nearby Attractions

The Shelton Laurel Backcountry has more trails that link to each other and the Appalachian Trail for multiple loop possibilities.

Directions

From Asheville, take I-26 north to Exit 19A/Marshall. From there, trace US 25/US 70 for 21 miles. Turn right (west) onto NC 208 and follow it 3.4 miles. Turn right (east) onto NC 212 and follow it 6.9 miles to reach Hickey Fork Road. There will be a sign indicating Shelton Laurel Backcountry. Turn left and follow Hickey Fork Road, which becomes FR 465 in the Pisgah National Forest, for 1.1 miles to a seasonally closed gate and parking area on your right.

7

Lovers Leap

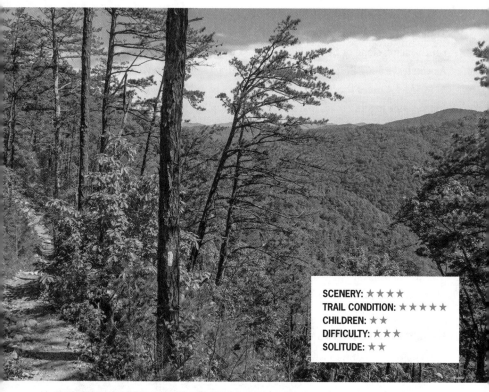

> SCENERY: ★ ★ ★ ★
> TRAIL CONDITION: ★ ★ ★ ★ ★
> CHILDREN: ★ ★
> DIFFICULTY: ★ ★ ★
> SOLITUDE: ★ ★

THIS PINE-BORDERED PART OF THE APPALACHIAN TRAIL STANDS HUNDREDS OF FEET ABOVE THE FRENCH BROAD RIVER.

TRAILHEAD GPS COORDINATES: 35.892570, -82.818489

DISTANCE & CONFIGURATION: 4.5-mile loop

HIKING TIME: 3 hours

HIGHLIGHTS: Views of the French Broad River and Hot Springs

ELEVATION: 1,314' along French Broad River, 2,382' on top of the ridge

ACCESS: Free and always open

MAPS: National Geographic #782 *French Broad and Nolichucky Rivers (Cherokee and Pisgah National Forests);* USGS *Hot Springs*

FACILITIES: None

WHEELCHAIR ACCESS: None

COMMENTS: This hike can be shortened by taking the Silvermine Trail from Lovers Leap back to the trailhead. (Or it can be considerably lengthened by continuing on the Appalachian Trail to Maine.)

CONTACTS: Pisgah National Forest, Appalachian Ranger District, 828-689-9694, fs.usda.gov/nfsnc

Overview

Nestled between the Blue Ridge Mountains and beside the French Broad River, the quaint town of Hot Springs anchors the Lovers Leap hike. The route follows the renowned Appalachian Trail (AT) beside the river and then presents a strenuous climb to Lovers Leap overlook. This rocky outcrop provides views of Hot Springs, the serpentine French Broad, and the distant ridgeline of the North Carolina–Tennessee border. Past Lovers Leap, the trail travels along the ridgeline before intersecting Pump Gap Trail. The route then follows Pump Gap Trail and weaves through the remnants of an old silver mining operation on its way back to the trailhead.

Route Details

You will begin the hike from a parking area up Silvermine Road, then walk it back down to join the Appalachian Trail directly beside the French Broad River, whose headwaters begin south of Asheville. However, because it falls to the west of the Eastern Continental Divide, the water flows north, traveling a winding route northwest through the mountains before emptying into the Tennessee River.

After backtracking down Silvermine Road to the French Broad River, look left for a small footbridge that spans Silvermine Creek. During summer, the creek is lined with Japanese knotweed, an invasive exotic species that now grows rampantly throughout the Southeast. Rising above the knotweed is a trailhead sign with a white blaze painted on it. Follow this marker across the footbridge that spans the creek, and then continue to follow the white blazes that lead south farther up the river.

As if this route weren't already confusing enough, when you literally hike south along the north-flowing river, you are theoretically progressing north on the most famous footpath in the world: the Appalachian Trail. The AT travels 2,198 miles from Georgia to Maine, and it is marked the entire way with the white blazes that you are now following alongside this river.

If you hike this trail in the spring, you may be passed from behind by several rugged, sometimes smelly thru-hikers who have set out to complete the entire trail in one calendar year. You may want to even consider bringing extra snacks in your day pack to share with these long-distance hikers. Sharing food along the AT is known as trail magic, and it is always appreciated.

Lovers Leap

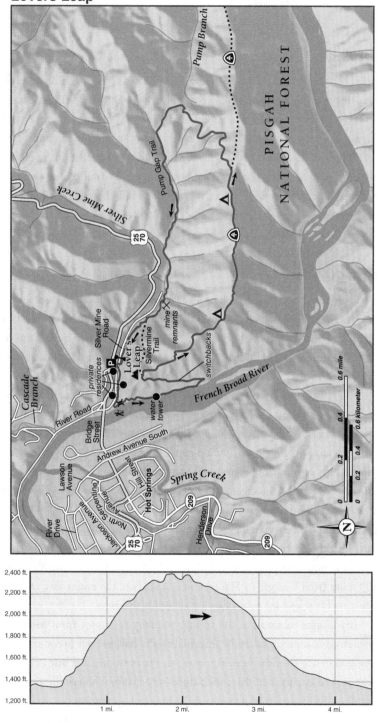

Along the river, you may spot purple wildflowers such as the funny-sounding beardtongue (a common name for penstemon) or tall-growing spiderwort. After 0.2 mile of hiking along the French Broad River, you will notice a concrete tower to your right. This tower once served to gauge the height of floodwaters on the French Broad. In another 0.2 mile the trail will take a sharp turn uphill. This is the first of many switchbacks that lead up the steep mountain. The multiple switchbacks will raise your heart rate, but after 0.3 mile your hard work will be rewarded with views from rock outcrops on either side of the final switchback.

The first rock outcrop is Lovers Leap, for which this route is named. Cherokee legend suggests that this rocky ledge was the site where the fair maiden Mist-of-the-Mountain threw herself off the mountain after she learned that her love had been murdered by a jealous rival. The next outcrop gives a better view back to Hot Springs and the French Broad River. This is also the trail junction with the Silvermine Trail. If you want to shorten your hike, you can take the Silvermine Trail down the mountain and arrive at the trailhead parking lot after 1.6 miles of total walking. Otherwise, remain on the AT and continue uphill.

The trail does not immediately flatten out but now climbs along the ridge of the mountain. In winter, the bare trees reveal views of neighboring mountains to the north and south. After 1.7 miles of cumulative hiking, you will reach a nice level campsite on the ridge. Continue on the rolling ridgeline of hardwood trees and mountain laurel thickets for another 1.3 miles to a second small campsite on the left of the trail. Just past this campsite, the AT intersects the blazed Pump Gap Trail. Turn left onto Pump Gap Trail and follow it downhill beside a small stream.

The next half mile gives the feeling of hiking through a long green tunnel. Lady ferns and doghobble choke the forest floor, while thick groves of rhododendrons and tall poplar trees flourish to your left and right.

After nearly a mile of descent, the Pump Gap Trail widens into an old roadbed. It continues to follow the stream down the valley and past the remnants of old bunkers, which were once used to hold explosives. I like to think that the sticks of dynamite have been removed, but the DANGER EXPLOSIVES sign keeps me from exploring the concrete shed too closely, and I recommend keeping a safe distance.

Continue on the old roadbed through a valley rife with wildflowers in spring, past the site of the old Silvermine Group Camp, then walk around the pole gate to reach the trailhead parking area.

Nearby Attractions

A visit to the town of Hot Springs can turn this 4.6-mile hike into a full day's outing. The main attraction is the Hot Springs Spa, where riverside hot tubs can be rented for an hour-long soak. These tubs are filled with water piped from the town's naturally occurring hot springs. After a relaxing dip in the tubs, be sure to satisfy your hiking hunger with a trip to one of the Spring Street restaurants serving delicious food. Also, don't leave town before visiting Bluff Mountain Outfitters. It's a wonderful store with a knowledgeable staff who can help you prepare for your next adventure.

Directions

From Asheville, travel US 19/US 23 north (future I-26) to Exit 19A. Turn left off the exit and follow US 25/US 70 west 25 miles. Just before crossing the bridge over the French Broad River and entering Hot Springs, turn right onto River Road. After 0.1 mile turn left onto Silvermine Road and travel underneath the overpass. Continue 0.3 mile to the parking area at the end of the road.

8 Bailey Mountain Preserve

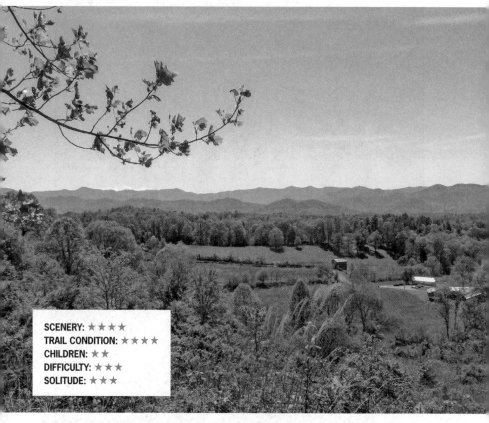

SCENERY: ★ ★ ★ ★
TRAIL CONDITION: ★ ★ ★ ★
CHILDREN: ★ ★
DIFFICULTY: ★ ★ ★
SOLITUDE: ★ ★ ★

THE PRESERVED SMITH FARM STANDS IN THE FOREGROUND, WITH THE BLUE RIDGE MOUNTAINS RISING BEYOND.

TRAILHEAD GPS COORDINATES: 35.843296, -82.559880

DISTANCE & CONFIGURATION: 5.3-mile balloon

HIKING TIME: 3 hours

HIGHLIGHTS: Views from meadows

ELEVATION: 2,410 feet at trailhead, 3,480 feet atop Bailey Mountain

ACCESS: No fees or permits required

MAPS: Bailey Mountain Preserve; USGS *Mars Hill*

FACILITIES: None

WHEELCHAIR ACCESS: None

CONTACTS: Town of Mars Hill, 828-689-2301, townofmarshill.org; libguides.mhu.edu/Bailey

Bailey Mountain Preserve

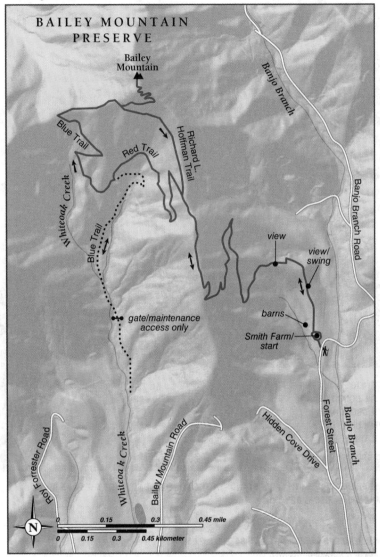

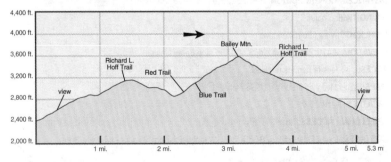

Overview

Discover this newer hiking destination near the town of Mars Hill. Start at the preserved Smith Farm, with its house, barns, and fields intact, then climb into woods, grabbing a pair of southward vistas before joining Connor Ridge. Begin the loop portion of the hike, dipping into the headwaters of Whiteoak Creek. Ascend to the wooded summit of Bailey Mountain, with limited views, before returning to the trailhead, savoring Western North Carolina farm and mountain history.

Route Details

As more and more people seek refuge in the mountain beauty of greater Asheville and Western North Carolina, so the pressure mounts to turn wooded mountain slopes into highland homes with views. And how can we blame others for wanting to live in such scenic places that we already call home? Yet we also know that it pays to preserve some places, whether to safeguard our collective farming history, or simply keep a beautiful mountain in a natural state. Bailey Mountain Preserve, a mere mile from the town of Mars Hill, does both. With the Smith Farm as an access to Bailey Mountain, an Appalachian mountain farm remains as it was for a century and a half, while a peak overlooking Mars Hills stays wild.

Opened in 2022, Bailey Mountain Preserve, over 250 acres strong, offers 6 miles of hiking trails to explore this peak looming above Mars Hill. Parts of the crown were timbered and some became pasture. Now we see places transitioning back to full-blown hardwood forest. The contiguous Smith Farm has undergone a multistage metamorphosis as well: from subsistence farm of the late 1800s to tobacco farm to cattle farm to preserved farmstead and trailhead—with plans of future enhancement for Bailey Mountain Preserve visitors.

The trail system—a combination of old farm roads and singletrack pathways—not only takes you to scenic sites but also challenges you with its vertical variation. The recommended 5.3-mile hike entails a net 1,500-foot elevation change, enough to get your legs and heart pumping. The trek begins at the parking area near the old Smith Farm farmhouse. A grassy track, the Richard L. Hoffman Trail, leads north, uphill, through preserved meadows that will display flowers in season, primarily late summer. Look back and enjoy the bucolic scene before entering the forest at 0.1 mile. Admire the huge old-growth oak tree with a wooden swing hanging from one of its prodigious limbs. If you can get away from the swing, continue climbing in woods via switchbacks, then come to a bench and grand overlook at 0.3 mile. Here, you can admire the nearby Smith Farm and Mars Hill. You can also see across the Ivy Creek Valley and onward to the Great Craggy Mountains and other ridges over which the Blue Ridge Parkway travels. No wonder this view needs a seat!

Continue the Richard L. Hoffman Trail, rising on a slope transitioning from field to forest. Switchbacks ease the ascent to Connor Ridge, which you make at 1.1 miles. From there, clamber northbound along the ridgeline and, at 1.5 miles, watch for the left turn at an intersection, where you join the Red Trail. This path switchbacks downhill, then circles the upper watershed of Whiteoak Creek, where you will step over rocky headwaters of the aforementioned stream, eventually dropping to a trail intersection at 2.1 miles. Here, you head right on

THIS ALLURING SWING MAY PROVE AN IMPEDIMENT TO YOUR PROGRESS.

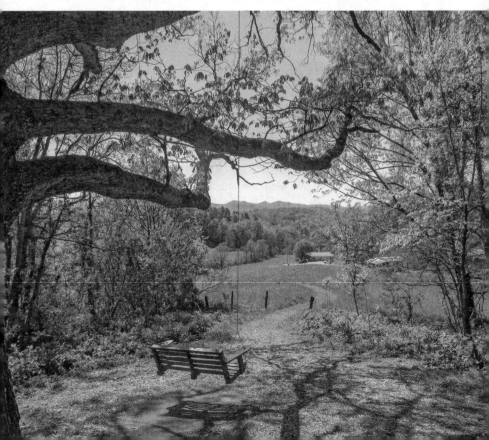

the Blue Trail, as it traces an old mountain road. The Blue Trail, heading left, descends to a property access open only to preserve management.

From this point you will climb 715 feet over the next mile. The Blue Trail makes the ascent more tolerable with switchbacks amid the rich forest. At 2.7 miles, your climb is rewarded by making Hamp Gap. You are now on the shoulder of Bailey Mountain, and more climbing lies ahead, but what's a mountain hike without a little climbing? Head east, working up the shoulder to make another trail intersection, at 2.9 miles, in a rocky section of Bailey Mountain. Turn left here, working uphill on a series of short switchbacks to top out at 3.2 miles. No stunning view awaits, just a winter look south to Mars Hill. Yet we can take satisfaction in climbing this preserved peak that holds a place in the array of highland splendor we call home.

Your hike back starts with a backtrack; then, at 3.5 miles, you head left on the Richard L. Hoffman Trail, relishing unabated downhill hiking, first running along Connor Ridge to finish the loop portion of the hike at 3.8 miles. From there, you stay with the Richard L. Hoffman Trail 1.5 miles back to the trailhead, enjoying the fair view a second time and perhaps reposing on the swing hanging from the massive oak tree that has seen what is now Bailey Mountain Preserve change through the decades.

Nearby Attractions

The town of Mars Hill and college of the same name are close to the trailhead for an easy visit.

Directions

From Asheville, take I-26 west to Exit 11, Mars Hill, then take NC 213 west/Carl Eller Road for 1 mile. Head right onto North Main Street and follow it 0.1 mile, then turn left onto Bailey Street and travel 0.3 mile. Turn left onto Hickory Drive, go 0.3 mile, then turn right onto Forest Street and drive 0.9 mile to reach the preserve trailhead on your left. Bailey Mountain Preserve address: 889 Forest Street, Mars Hill, NC.

Rattlesnake Lodge

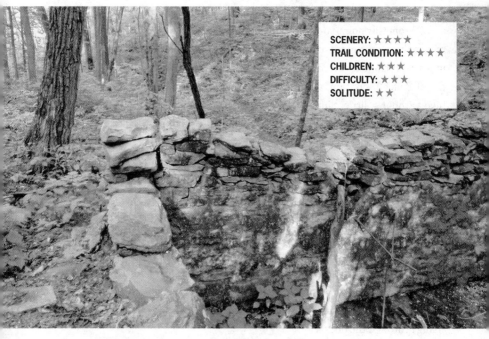

SCENERY: ★ ★ ★ ★
TRAIL CONDITION: ★ ★ ★ ★
CHILDREN: ★ ★ ★
DIFFICULTY: ★ ★ ★
SOLITUDE: ★ ★

ROCK FOUNDATIONS BORDER THE TRAIL AT RATTLESNAKE LODGE.

TRAILHEAD GPS COORDINATES: 35.669727, -82.471227

DISTANCE & CONFIGURATION: 3.8-mile balloon

HIKING TIME: 2.5 hours

HIGHLIGHTS: Rock ruins of Dr. Chase P. Ambler's early 1900s mountain retreat

ELEVATION: 3,165' at trailhead, 4,050' at the main spring

ACCESS: Free and always open. If the Blue Ridge Parkway is closed, you can still access the trailhead from Ox Creek Road in Weaverville or Elk Mountain Road in Asheville.

MAPS: National Geographic #779 *Linville Gorge, Mount Mitchell;* USGS *Craggy Pinnacle*

FACILITIES: None

WHEELCHAIR ACCESS: None

COMMENTS: Rattlesnake Lodge is also accessible via a 0.4-mile side trail marked by blue blazes. That route may be preferable for families with very small children or for hikers with limited time. Parking for this alternate trail is located just north of Tanbark Ridge Tunnel on the Blue Ridge Parkway (Trailhead GPS Coordinates: 35.665666, -82.461847) .

CONTACTS: Blue Ridge Parkway, 828-298-0398, nps.gov/blri; Mountains-to-Sea Trail, 919-825-0297, mountainstosea.org

Overview

More than 100 years ago, Rattlesnake Lodge was a private summer destination for prominent Asheville doctor and conservationist Chase P. Ambler, his family, and friends. Today the rock ruins that remain offer unique appeal for area hikers. The Rattlesnake Lodge route follows the Mountains-to-Sea Trail (MST) to the foundations of Dr. Ambler's summer home, swimming pool, shed, and reservoir. Pausing at the onetime Ambler property, it's not hard to imagine the family spending a hot July day soaking in the pool or watching a mountain sunset from their front porch. The rockwork alone serves as a reward, even when rain or fog hides the mountain views.

Route Details

Access the trail to Rattlesnake Lodge from a small dirt pullout along Ox Creek Road. To begin the hike, walk just past the boulders that separate the parking area from the forest. Then turn left onto the MST, which itself spans more than 1,175 miles in North Carolina—from Great Smoky Mountains National Park to the Outer Banks. The balloon hike to Rattlesnake Lodge showcases more than 2 miles of this wonderful North Carolina resource.

Walk uphill, following the round, white MST blazes. The next 0.6 mile of trail features some of the finest switchbacks in the Southeast. The trail winds upward on a gentle grade through a hardwood forest and amid heavy undergrowth in the summer months. In late spring, a variety of wildflowers borders the trail and brings a rainbow of bright colors to the dense green underbrush. Consider bringing a wildflower book to identify beauties such as white-fringed phacelia, fire pink fuchsia, and purple spiderwort.

When the switchbacks cease, the path veers east and continues its mild elevation gain toward Rattlesnake Lodge. Several good spots along this stretch beckon you to stop and catch your breath. In spring, look for heavy pockets of flaming azaleas. Year-round breaks in the canopy reveal views of the Swannanoa River Valley to the south. After hiking a mile, reach an opening in the trees that provides a glimpse of triangular-shaped Lane Pinnacle looming to the east. (If you were to continue past Rattlesnake Lodge for several miles, the MST would take you to the top of this mountain.)

Rattlesnake Lodge

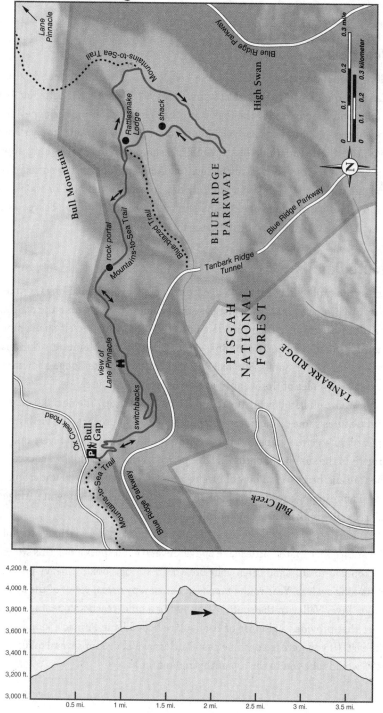

Large boulders on either side of the trail signify the 1.2-mile mark. These two pillars serve as a rock portal to Rattlesnake Lodge. From this point, the trail levels out and you may begin to notice moss-covered remains of a rock wall poking up through the leaf cover to your right.

After 1.5 miles of hiking, you will arrive at the ruins of Dr. Ambler's summer retreat. While only the stone foundations of the lodge and outer buildings exist today, Dr. Ambler's legacy lives on. He was a founder of the Appalachian Mountain Club, from which the Carolina Mountain Club spun off. The Carolina Mountain Club is currently the most active hiking and trail maintenance organization in Asheville. Interestingly, club members maintain the MST near Dr. Ambler's Rattlesnake Lodge.

Upon approaching the ruins, the first major landmark you will see is the leaf-filled swimming pool to the right. After that, the trail comes to a level plateau that juts into the forest. A century ago, this level site was used for the main lodge and the courtyard; today it houses a fire ring and several prime camping spots.

At this point, you may be curious about the background of this place. According to the National Park Service, Rattlesnake Lodge received its name (after it was built) from the multiple rattlesnake skins that adorned the ceiling in the property's living room. Dr. Ambler was said to pay $5 for each rattlesnake, and reports suggest that more than 40 of the tan-and-brown reptiles were killed in the first three summers at the lodge. (The website suggests that, in those days, $5 was equivalent to one week's wages.) In 1920 Dr. Ambler sold his lodge, and in 1926 the building burned down, most likely due to lightning.

The structure must have been susceptible to fire, as Dr. Ambler had ordered that his summer home be built with sturdy chestnut wood from local trees. At that time, chestnut trees were plentiful in the southern Appalachian Mountains. Unfortunately, in the following decades the chestnut tree population was decimated by an invasive blight. Today, along the side of the trail, you may notice several chestnut saplings, but these young trees will likely live only for a few years before the invasive fungus overcomes them.

Continuing on the MST, reach an intersection with a blue-blazed trail just before the substantial remains of Dr. Ambler's toolshed. Turn left on the blue-blazed trail past the springhouse and begin a strenuous climb. After 0.2 mile of heart-pounding, uphill hiking, you will pass Rattlesnake Lodge's main water reservoir. Continue another 0.2 mile to the homestead's primary spring. At the main spring, the blue-blazed trail rejoins the MST. Having climbed nearly 2 miles after leaving the spring, you will follow a gently sloping downhill for the remainder of the hike.

Turn right and follow the white blazes through a long mountain laurel tunnel that loops back toward the lodge. These mountain laurels flower into a beautiful pink-and-white roof for hikers to walk underneath during the month of June. However, if you stand more than 6 feet tall, you may find yourself ducking to avoid some of the branches.

After hiking 2.2 miles, you will come to a well-preserved stone chimney that was part of the Amblers' so-called shack. The shack, next to a small stream, was home to a water-driven generator that provided electricity to the lodge.

At 2.4 miles, just before completing the upper loop, pass the blue-blazed spur dropping left to the trailhead near Tanbark Ridge Tunnel. Beyond the intersection, continue to follow the MST and retrace your steps downhill, zig-zagging multiple switchbacks, to arrive back at the trailhead parking lot off Ox Creek Road.

Directions

From downtown Asheville, drive east on College Street toward Tunnel Road. At the traffic light before Beaucatcher Tunnel, turn left onto Town Mountain Road. Carefully follow the winding turns on Town Mountain Road for 6.5 miles to Craven Gap, where Town Mountain Road dead-ends at the Blue Ridge Parkway. There, turn left and travel the Blue Ridge Parkway north 1 mile to reach Ox Creek Road. Turn left on Ox Creek Road and follow it 0.8 mile, past Elk Mountain Road to the left and a small gravel pullout to the right. Just before Ox Creek Road takes a sharp left turn, there is a dirt parking lot to the right: this is the Rattlesnake Lodge Trailhead.

Hawkbill Rock

SCENERY: ★ ★ ★ ★ ★
TRAIL CONDITION: ★ ★ ★
CHILDREN: ★ ★ ★
DIFFICULTY: ★ ★ ★ ★
SOLITUDE: ★ ★ ★ ★ ★

GAZING UP TOWARD THE CREST OF THE BLUE RIDGE FROM HAWKBILL ROCK

TRAILHEAD GPS COORDINATES: 35.699987, -82.398871

DISTANCE & CONFIGURATION: 2.8-mile out-and-back

HIKING TIME: 2 hours

HIGHLIGHTS: Outstanding views from Hawkbill Rock

ELEVATION: 4,917' at trailhead, 5,374' on top of Snowball Mountain

ACCESS: Free, but vehicle access to this hike is unavailable when the Blue Ridge Parkway is closed. Check nps.gov/blri for real-time road closures.

MAPS: National Geographic #779 *Linville Gorge, Mount Mitchell;* USGS *Craggy Pinnacle*

FACILITIES: Picnic tables, outdoor grills, and restrooms at Craggy Gardens Picnic Area

WHEELCHAIR ACCESS: None

COMMENTS: This hike can be lengthened by walking 1.7 miles past Hawkbill Rock to Little Snowball Mountain. However, if you plan to journey past Hawkbill Rock, bring a good map, as the trail is lesser used.

CONTACTS: Blue Ridge Parkway, 828-298-0398, nps.gov/blri

Hawkbill Rock

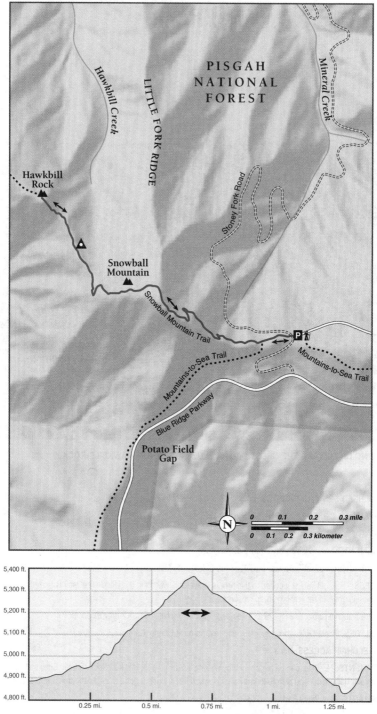

Overview

This trail starts near the entrance of the Craggy Gardens Picnic Area and follows the Mountains-to-Sea Trail (MST) briefly before veering north on the Snowball Mountain Trail. There is a short but difficult climb to the top of Snowball Mountain, followed by a moderate descent along the peak's narrow ridge. The highlight of the hike is the dramatic view from Hawkbill Rock. However, you must first overcome a challenging but enjoyable rock scramble in order to access the scenic outcrop.

Route Details

Look for the trailhead before a park gate that leads to Craggy Gardens Picnic Area. It is located at a 90-degree bend in the road, near roadside parking and to the left of a dirt turnoff for Stoney Fork Road.

Begin the hike by following the white-blazed MST west and slightly uphill. After 0.1 mile the singletrack trail will split in two. The white-blazed MST continues on the left toward Lane Pinnacle, and the yellow-blazed Snowball Mountain Trail veers right. Take the less-traveled Snowball Mountain Trail. Because this path does not receive as much foot traffic as other trails in the area, there may be heavy underbrush encroaching upon the narrow dirt treadway. If you are hiking this route in the summer or fall, it is a good idea to wear long pants in order to protect your legs from stray thorns, nettles, and poison ivy.

After departing the MST, start a set of switchbacks leading to the summit of Snowball Mountain. The steady incline offers a short but challenging 0.5-mile climb. The top of Snowball Mountain is covered with oak, beech, and yellow birch trees. Catch glimpses of neighboring mountains from atop Snowball Mountain, but know that the best views are revealed in November when the leaves have fallen.

If the parkway remains open late into the season, and you are able to hike this trail after peak leaf season, then you will have an easy time identifying the beech trees. Beech trees have leaves that are marcescent, meaning that they do not naturally detach in autumn and, instead, stay on the tree until strong winds, rains, or heavy snow cause them to fall. Their translucent brown hue often glimmers in shades of copper and gold when the winter sun pierces through the bare canopy of the forest.

Descending the northwest spine of Snowball Mountain, you will continue through a dense hardwood forest that exhibits some relatively mature chestnut trees (up to 10 feet tall). *Relative* is the key word because chestnut trees rarely live more than a few years due to the deadly chestnut blight. You may also recognize a few buckeye trees lining the path or discover their shiny brown-and-tan fruit lining the trail in autumn.

Once you have hiked 1 mile, you will reach what seems to be a modest viewpoint. However, one step up onto a neighboring rock will allow you to see over the shrubs and out across Big Fork Ridge, Bullhead Ridge, and Locust Ridge to the north. After leaving the overlook, continue downhill to a nearby gap. Upon reaching the brief dip in the ridgeline, you will face your final ascent to Hawkbill Rock. This last climb will force you to do some rock scrambling as the soft earthen path transitions into angled granite.

You will have to use both of your hands and both of your feet to navigate this steep, exposed section. And although your eyes will be focused on the trail,

EASTERLY VIEW TOWARD CRAGGY PINNACLE

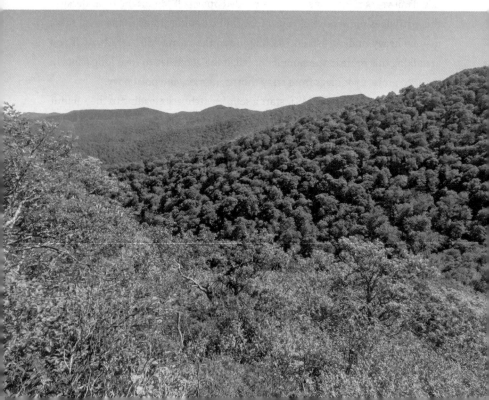

be sure to look to your left, as the main outcrop of Hawkbill Rock is hidden from the path. The best way to find this majestic viewpoint, located 1.3 miles from the start of the trail, is to stop hiking just before the trail reenters the forest. There is a slight rise in the granite rock to your left. If you take a few steps over to this rise, you will be able to look below and see the smooth rock slab known as Hawkbill Rock. Carefully navigate down to this overlook and enjoy the fantastic view of Reems Creek Valley.

Tributaries running off the side of Snowball Mountain and Rocky Knob create Reems Creek, which wanders about 20 miles through the fertile valley below before ending at the French Broad River. This region was one of the first areas of Western North Carolina to be settled by Europeans. It also was the birthplace of Zebulon Vance, a North Carolina governor, US senator, and Confederate leader during the Civil War.

When you are ready to leave Hawkbill Rock, backtrack to the trailhead on the Snowball Mountain Trail.

Nearby Attractions

The Craggy Gardens Picnic Area, at the end of Craggy Garden Picnic Area Road, offers picnic tables, outdoor grills, and restroom facilities.

Directions

From Asheville follow the Blue Ridge Parkway north to mile marker 367.5 and turn left onto Craggy Gardens Picnic Area Road. The closest parking to the trailhead is located off the side of the Craggy Gardens Picnic Area Road, at a sharp right turn and just before a park gate. If there are not available spaces alongside the road, continue to the main parking and picnic area and begin your hike by backtracking alongside the road.

Douglas Falls

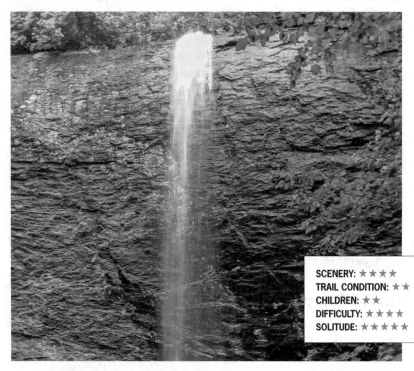

SCENERY: ★ ★ ★ ★
TRAIL CONDITION: ★ ★
CHILDREN: ★ ★
DIFFICULTY: ★ ★ ★ ★
SOLITUDE: ★ ★ ★ ★ ★

THE SHEER WHITE CURTAIN OF DOUGLAS FALLS DIVES PAST AN IMPOSING STONE FACE.

TRAILHEAD GPS COORDINATES: 35.700250, -82.379600

DISTANCE & CONFIGURATION: 6.6-mile out-and-back

HIKING TIME: 4 hours

HIGHLIGHTS: 70-foot Douglas Falls

ELEVATION: 5,490' at trailhead, 4,218' at Douglas Falls

ACCESS: Free, but vehicle access to this hike is unavailable when the Blue Ridge Parkway is closed. Check nps.gov/blri for real-time road closures.

MAPS: National Geographic #779 *Linville Gorge, Mount Mitchell*; USGS *Craggy Pinnacle*

FACILITIES: Restrooms and water at Craggy Gardens Visitor Center

WHEELCHAIR ACCESS: Yes, at the Craggy Gardens Visitor Center

COMMENTS: For children and adults who may not want to hike the 6.6 miles round-trip from the parkway, you can also reach Douglas Falls from a 0.5-mile trail near Barnardsville. (See "Directions" for the time-consuming and bumpy drive to the trailhead for the shorter hike.)

CONTACTS: Blue Ridge Parkway, 828-298-0398, nps.gov/blri; Pisgah National Forest, 828-257-4200, fs.usda.gov/nfsnc

Overview

The trail to Douglas Falls weaves steadily downhill through a dense hardwood forest. After you turn off the Mountains-to-Sea Trail (MST), you will not cross another trail intersection or road on your journey to the falls, making this a very quiet and remote hike. You will cross several streams before reaching a grove of large boulders and a 70-foot-long rock ledge. The slender but picturesque Douglas Falls drops over the ledge into a small pool. After leaving the waterfall, the hike back to the trailhead presents an unrelenting uphill climb. It is imperative that you allow ample daylight time for completing this hike, particularly because of the tiring uphill climb on the return leg.

Route Details

The Blue Ridge Parkway attracts an estimated 16 million people each year, according to the National Park Service. However, only a small fraction of those visitors know about Douglas Falls, a hidden jewel located near milepost 364.

Parking for Douglas Falls is on either side of the Craggy Gardens Visitor Center. To begin the hike, follow the paved sidewalk at the visitor center southeast toward Craggy Gardens. When the sidewalk reaches the forest, it turns into a dirt path that quickly leads to the MST, which is blazed with white circles. At the junction with the MST, it is important to turn right and follow the MST and Douglas Falls signs to the north. (A left turn will lead up the hill to the Craggy Gardens Pavilion.)

The next 1 mile of trail is fairly level but very rocky. Your feet will land on the hard jagged rocks that cover the trail far more often than the patches of soft dirt that sporadically appear. This section can be especially precarious if the rocks are slick. Wearing proper hiking footwear will help give you traction over the coarse terrain, but you may also want to consider bringing a hiking stick or two to help with balance.

After hiking a cumulative 1.2 miles, leave the MST and veer left onto the Douglas Falls Trail. This path is not as well traveled as the MST and can become overgrown in the summer and early fall. From this point forward, you will follow yellow rectangular blazes on a steady descent to Douglas Falls. Thankfully, the route includes several switchbacks, so the downhill grade is never too steep. Do not take the cut-off trails that shorten the switchbacks. If you were to take

Douglas Falls

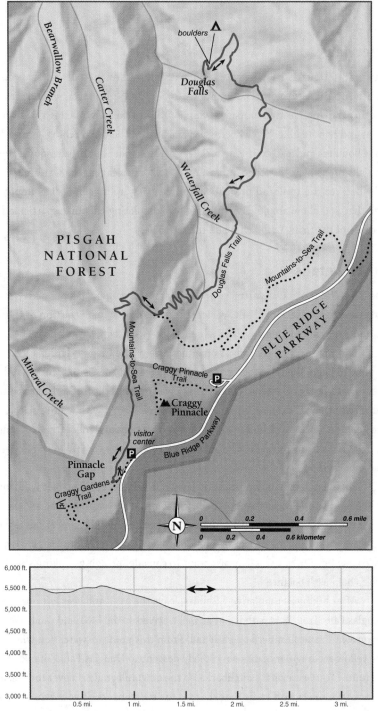

these shortcuts, you would contribute to erosion, create a new and often confusing trail, and detract from the trail's gradual climb. In fact, it is a Leave No Trace principle to walk only on established trails, so do your best to stay on the official pathway!

At 1.7 miles the trail crosses Waterfall Creek. Because the stream cascades for a considerable distance above and below the trail, hikers will sometimes mistake this small stream for Douglas Falls. It is NOT Douglas Falls, but it can be quite a sight when robustly flowing. Use caution when crossing this slick streambed. You still have 1.6 miles to go to reach the waterfall.

Beyond Waterfall Creek the trail can become more overgrown. During spring beautiful trillium plants carpet the path, but in late summer the trilliums thicken with stinging nettles. In the Southern Appalachians, these nettles can grow up to 4 feet tall and are characterized by their opposite leaves with serrated edges. If you fail to recognize the plants by sight, then you will most likely identify them due to the stinging sensation from grazing against the plant. Instinctively, you will want to rub or scratch at the invisible irritation, but the more you touch it, the worse it can become. Typically, the burning and itching caused by a stinging nettle will fade away within 15 minutes, but if it persists, you may want to apply cold water and hydrocortisone cream. Or, better yet, you can wear long pants to avoid contact with the nettle.

Meanwhile, the path continues down the mountain and seemingly deeper into the woods. The lower the elevation and the farther from the parkway that you hike, the quieter the woods will become. There is no noise pollution on the lower half of this trail, and the woods along the path reveal a setting that seems timeless. You can envision someone standing in these woods 1,000 years ago and surveying a similar scene to what you witness today. Because of the remote location and solitude on this trail, it is advisable to never hike this route alone—and never count on smartphone reception on any hike, but particularly one as isolated as this.

At 3.2 miles reach two large boulders and a backcountry campsite. Go to the right of the second boulder and follow a long switchback to reach Douglas Falls. The amount of water coming over the falls is minimal compared with other waterfalls in the area, but the steep 70-foot drop and dramatic rock cliff make this an unforgettable destination. It is possible to walk behind and around the falls or to stand directly under it—if you can tolerate the cold water—but be careful on and around the slick rocks, as it's easy to lose your balance and fall.

Be mentally prepared for the long uphill journey back to the trailhead. Most out-and-back hikes gain elevation in the first half of the hike. This trail often feels more difficult because you must climb 1,000 feet in the second half of the hike. Take your time and, as noted above, begin your hike in time to allow for plenty of daylight for your ascent back to the parking lot.

Nearby Attractions

The trail starts and ends at the Craggy Gardens Visitor Center off the Blue Ridge Parkway. At the visitor center you can view maps, talk to the knowledgeable staff, and purchase parkway gifts.

Directions

Take the Blue Ridge Parkway north from Asheville. Drive to milepost 364, approximately 18 miles from Asheville, and park at the Craggy Gardens Visitor Center to the left of the parkway.

If you prefer the shorter version of this hike to Douglas Falls (see "Comments," page 70), drive this route: from Barnardsville, follow Dillingham Road 6 miles to reach Forest Road 74. Travel 8.7 miles on FR 74 to the Douglas Falls trailhead.

12 Craggy Gardens and Craggy Pinnacle

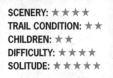

SCENERY: ★ ★ ★ ★
TRAIL CONDITION: ★ ★
CHILDREN: ★ ★
DIFFICULTY: ★ ★ ★ ★
SOLITUDE: ★ ★ ★ ★ ★

A VIEW OF THE BLUE RIDGE PARKWAY FROM CRAGGY PINNACLE

TRAILHEAD GPS COORDINATES (CRAGGY GARDENS VISITOR CENTER): 35.699709, -82.379929

TRAILHEAD GPS COORDINATES (CRAGGY PINNACLE PARKING): 35.704617, -82.373837

DISTANCE & CONFIGURATION: Two separate but nearby, 1-mile out-and-backs (not counting car shuttle)

HIKING TIME: 1.5 hours

HIGHLIGHTS: Panoramic views and blooming rhododendrons

ELEVATION: 5,481' at the visitor center, 5,877' at Craggy Pinnacle

ACCESS: Free, but vehicle access to this hike is unavailable when the Blue Ridge Parkway is closed. Check nps.gov/blri for real-time road closures.

MAPS: National Geographic #779 *Linville Gorge, Mount Mitchell;* USGS *Craggy Pinnacle*

FACILITIES: Restrooms and water at the Craggy Gardens Visitor Center

WHEELCHAIR ACCESS: Yes, at the visitor center

COMMENTS: Combine two neighboring trails to complete this hike, with a brief car shuttle to connect the hikes.

CONTACTS: Blue Ridge Parkway, 828-298-0398, nps.gov/blri

Craggy Gardens and Craggy Pinnacle

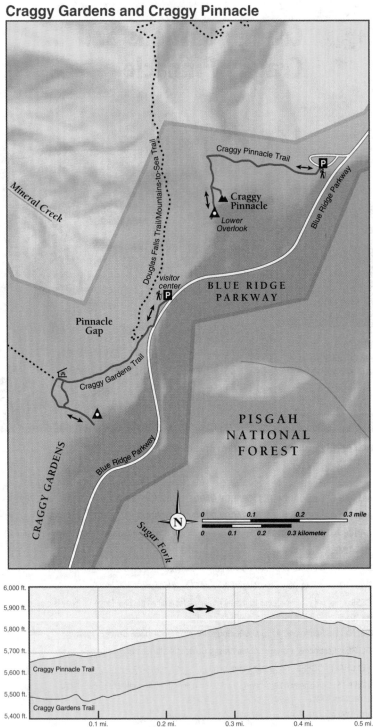

Overview

The Great Craggy Mountains feature the closest balds to Asheville, and those mountain summits reveal some of the best views in Western North Carolina. This combo hike will take you on two short out-and-back trails. On the first segment, you will follow the Mountains-to-Sea Trail (MST) to the rhododendron-dotted summit at Craggy Gardens. Then, after a short car shuttle, the second portion of the hike sends you to the top of Craggy Pinnacle for panoramic views of the North Fork Reservoir and neighboring Craggy Dome.

Route Details

Begin at the Craggy Gardens Visitor Center. Before starting your hike, consider spending time at the visitor center to learn more about the Craggy Gardens area, view a local map, and talk to the knowledgeable attendant working at the parkway store.

When you leave the visitor center, head southwest along the paved sidewalk to the end of the car park. There the sidewalk terminates and becomes a dirt spur trail leading into the forest. Turn right on the trail and follow it 0.1 mile to an intersection with Douglas Falls Trail and the MST. Turn left and hike uphill on the white-blazed MST. You will immediately notice the first of five informational plaques to your left. Each of the plaques that line the path to Craggy Gardens reveals a fascinating fact about the surrounding habitat.

The trail leading to the top of the mountain is a dark-green tunnel of birch, ash, oak, and buckeye trees. The trail is canopied so well that it comes as a surprise when you suddenly step out of the tree cover into the open air at Craggy Gardens. The first thing you will see on the bald is the large open-air pavilion. This is a great place to picnic or share a quick snack before exploring the bald.

Many scientists debate how the mountaintop balds first appeared in this region. One theory suggests that the balds were left after devastating wildfires destroyed mountaintop vegetation. Other researchers believe that balds were created by American Indians to attract certain animals. Today, the forest service maintains the balds via controlled burns or livestock grazing.

When you are ready to venture out onto the bald, walk to the south end of the pavilion and follow a maintained, but unmarked, trail to the left. This trail wanders across the exposed bald and through the low-lying shrubs that grow sparsely on the mountain. At the east end of the bald, the path terminates at a rock outcrop. On a clear day this vista provides stunning views of the North Fork drainage basin, Mount Graybeard, and the Black Mountains. By retracing your steps and taking the first available right, you can complete a loop on the bald and return to the Craggy Gardens Pavilion.

To access the next (Craggy Pinnacle) portion of this hike, you will need to backtrack to the Craggy Gardens Visitor Center and then drive your car north on the parkway for 1 mile through the Craggy Pinnacle Tunnel to the Craggy Dome viewing area and park in the lot on the left. The hike begins at the upper portion of the parking lot.

Before heading into the forest on the singletrack trail, take a minute to scan north for Craggy Dome. At 6,105 feet, Craggy Dome is the tallest peak in the Great Craggy Mountains.

The ascent to Craggy Pinnacle starts gradually and increases in difficulty as you approach the summit. A tunnel of rhododendron branches covers the first part of the trail. Both Craggy Gardens and Craggy Pinnacle are known for their early summer explosion of rhododendron blossoms. The pink and purple flowers start to bloom in early to mid-June and typically last until July.

At 0.2 mile the rhododendrons give way to wind-stunted birch trees, and you will notice several intriguing root formations that line the trail. The gnarled trees seemingly grow out of rocks, and each protruding root formation has its own unique features and shape. For the next 100 yards, the twisted exhibition lines the trail like pieces of art in a museum.

Beyond the peculiar birch trees, you will pass a seasonal spring on the left, and the grade of the trail will increase. At 0.3 mile you will arrive at a trail junction that divides the upper summit from the lower overlook. Veer left and travel another few hundred yards to the upper summit. The 360-degree views from the top of the mountain showcase Craggy Dome to the north and Craggy Gardens to the south. On the east side of the mountain, you can see the North Fork Reservoir, Asheville's water source, at the base of the Black Mountain range. To the west stand Mount Pisgah, Black Balsam Knob, and Cold Mountain; on a very clear day you may be able to pick out the faint ridge of the Great Smoky Mountains.

When you leave the summit, backtrack down the trail, but don't return to the trailhead before first turning left on the short side trail to the lower overlook. There, once again, great views spread forth to the south and east, and you are able to observe large, exposed rocks jutting out from the side of the mountain. After taking one last look at Craggy Gardens in front of you and Craggy Pinnacle above you, enjoy the short jaunt down the mountain to reach the trailhead and return to your car.

Directions

For part one of this two-pronged hike, take the Blue Ridge Parkway north from Asheville. Drive to milepost 364, approximately 18 miles from Asheville, and park at the Craggy Gardens Visitor Center to the left of the parkway. As noted above, for part two of the outing, drive 1 mile north on the parkway to the Craggy Dome viewing area and park in the lot on the left.

A MAINTAINED BUT UNMARKED TRAIL WANDERS THROUGH THE CRAGGY GARDENS.

East

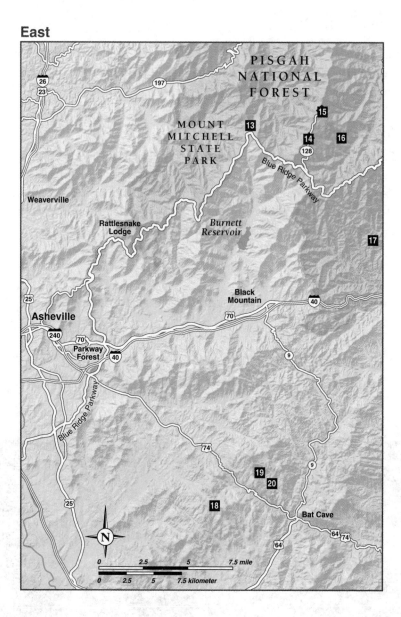

East

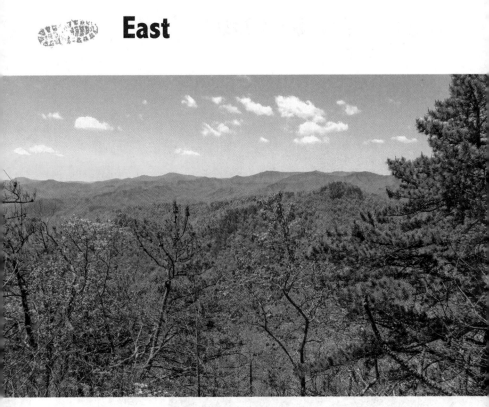

A HIKE TO SNOOKS NOSE DELIVERS VIEWS LIKE THIS (Hike 17, page 102).

Big Butt Little Butt

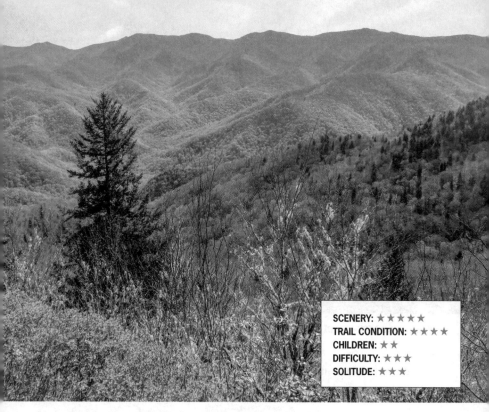

SCENERY: ★ ★ ★ ★ ★
TRAIL CONDITION: ★ ★ ★ ★
CHILDREN: ★ ★
DIFFICULTY: ★ ★ ★
SOLITUDE: ★ ★ ★

MOUNT MITCHELL AND THE BLACK MOUNTAINS AS SEEN FROM THE BIG BUTT TRAIL

TRAILHEAD GPS COORDINATES: 35.748508, -82.333910

DISTANCE & CONFIGURATION: 6.4-mile out-and-back

HIKING TIME: 3.2 hours

HIGHLIGHTS: Views from Little Butt and Big Butt, spruce forest, entire hike stays above a mile high

ELEVATION: 5,310' at trailhead, 5,948' atop Big Butt

ACCESS: No fees or permits required

MAPS: National Geographic #779 *Pisgah National Forest: Linville Gorge Mount Mitchell*; USGS *Mount Mitchell*

FACILITIES: None

WHEELCHAIR ACCESS: None

CONTACTS: Pisgah National Forest, 828-689-9694, fs.usda.gov/nfsnc

Overview

This hike starts and stays over a mile high, wandering out Brush Fence Ridge over Point Misery to Little Butt and an open outcrop presenting a first-rate view of Mount Mitchell and the Black Mountain Range. From there, continue toward Big Butt, capping your hike off with a peak bag of Big Butt and a distant view to the north and west.

Route Details

When you are literally one ridge over from North Carolina's fabled Black Mountains, where Mount Mitchell soars higher than every other peak east of the Mississippi River, you tend to be forgotten, a second fiddle mountain. However, Brush Fence Ridge, running parallel to the Black Mountains, offers a fine hike over three peaks, one of which presents a grandstand viewing platform of the mountains—where those majestic highlands stand out in brash relief. The trail to this grandstand is the Big Butt Trail, named for the highest of the three peaks you will visit, standing a shade under 6,000 feet. The path is in fine shape and exudes the high-country aura found where fragrant spruce spread their resiny perfume among gnarled yellow birch and beech, where a grassy understory waves in a cool breeze. It's a place where scattered outcrops rise as gray battlements in the forest, where the highland drops away to Ivy Creek and the Cane River, and where you can find repose in sterling natural splendor.

The hike starts at the Walker Knob Overlook on the Blue Ridge Parkway, at Balsam Gap. Locate and join the Big Butt Trail, heading northwest to briefly run along the parkway. Avoid the Mountains-to-Sea Trail that crosses the parkway here, as well as the old Wilson Boundary jeep road (not shown on the map). Once you're on the singletrack Big Butt Trail, scamper under yellow birch and spruce with a surprising number of red trilliums, also known as wake robins, as well as scads of lily-of-the-valley. At 0.1 mile, join Brush Fence Ridge, turning northbound with national forest property to your left and private property to the right, though the scenery is the same. Roll along the ridge; then, at 0.5 mile, the first set of wooden stairs eases you up a steep, narrow, craggy section, wreathed in rhododendrons. Shortly top out on a knob, then dip to a gap before making the steady but moderate ascent to 5,715-foot Point Misery, which you reach by a short spur at 1.5 miles. The wooded peak with no views is

Big Butt Little Butt

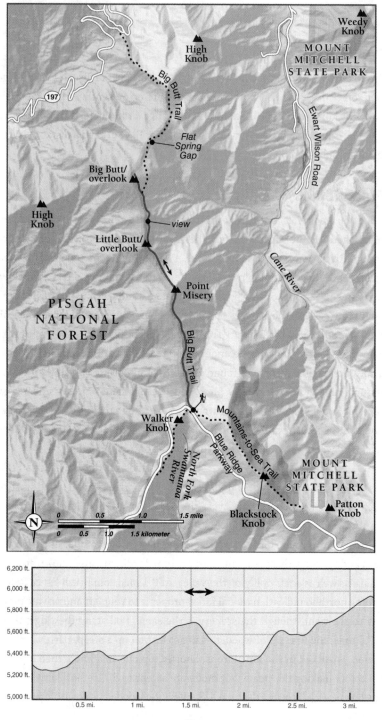

duly noted by a survey marker, and there has been a geocache here in the past. The reason for the name has been lost to time, but you can wager the moniker had something to do with the cold, wind, rain, and/or snow that often assaults these highest mantles outside of Asheville. This particular ridge also forms the boundary between Buncombe and Yancey Counties.

From Point Misery, the Big Butt Trail descends in switchbacks down a sharp mountain slope, dropping 350 feet in the next half mile. Wooden steps assist your descent. Little Butt rises in the yon. Bottom out in a wildflower-rich gap, then enter an area of great stone protuberances. Trace a magnificent piece of trail work rising among pillars, weaving between the steep rocks. At 2.3 miles, atop Little Butt, split right on a spur trail leading to an open rock face stretched east across the Cane River to Mount Mitchell and the peaks of the Black Mountains. What a view! You can also gander north down the Cane River Valley. This is a chance to relax and relish this grandstand of Mount Mitchell. The views are best in the afternoon, when a westering sun illuminates the mountains.

Beyond the view, the Big Butt Trail leads past a small campsite, then makes another relatively short climb (the highest single uptick on this entire hike is a mere 360 feet over 0.7 mile) along the slender ridge, parts of which are bordered in wind-stunted laurel. At 3.0 miles, reach an intersection. Here, the more heavily used and signed Big Butt Summit Trail splits left, while the Big Butt Trail descends a half mile to Flat Spring Gap and a campsite with an accessible spring, then beyond NC 197 at Cane River Gap. Stay left with the Big Butt Summit Trail, passing a small dry campsite, then continuing upward among wind-stunted hardwoods. Reach the peak of Big Butt, 5,948 feet, at 3.2 miles, as noted by a survey marker. And speaking of survey, trace the spur left to survey a cleared overlook (hopefully still cleared when you are there) that extends views north and west. Look for I-26 coursing north for Tennessee. I've been here on a clear day and picked out individual peaks in the Smokies 50 miles away! Enjoy the walk back to the trailhead, as it entails more down than up, as well as plenty of scenery worth a second look.

Nearby Attractions

The Blue Ridge Parkway presents nearly limitless outdoor attractions, and Mount Mitchell State Park stands but a few miles away, the entrance of which is less than 4 miles from this trailhead, milepost 355.4.

Directions

From Asheville, take the Blue Ridge Parkway north for 23 miles to the Walker Knob Overlook, milepost 358.9.

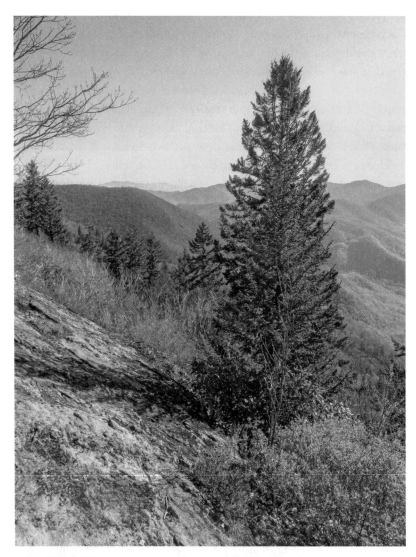

A VIEW FROM BRUSH FENCE RIDGE INTO THE CANE RIVER VALLEY

Mount Mitchell
High Loop

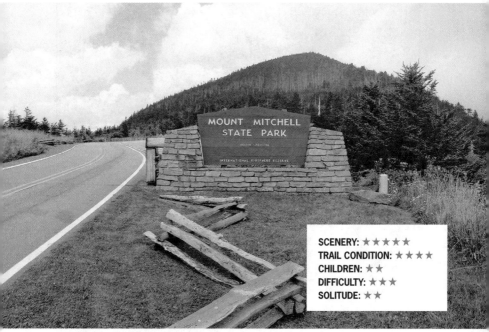

SCENERY: ★ ★ ★ ★ ★
TRAIL CONDITION: ★ ★ ★ ★
CHILDREN: ★ ★
DIFFICULTY: ★ ★ ★
SOLITUDE: ★ ★

WELCOME TO MOUNT MITCHELL STATE PARK.

TRAILHEAD GPS COORDINATES: 35.752662, -82.273731

DISTANCE & CONFIGURATION: 4-mile loop

HIKING TIME: 2.5 hours

HIGHLIGHTS: Mount Mitchell, the tallest mountain east of the Mississippi River

ELEVATION: 6,072' at trailhead, 6,684' at Mount Mitchell summit

ACCESS: May be limited in winter due to Blue Ridge Parkway closures. Check nps.gov/blri for real-time closures.

MAPS: Mount Mitchell State Park; USGS *Mount Mitchell*

FACILITIES: Restrooms and park information at the trailhead; restrooms, gift shop, and snack bar 0.2 mile beneath the summit

WHEELCHAIR ACCESS: Yes, on a 0.2-mile trail from the upper parking lot to the summit

COMMENTS: This hike is rated for moderate distance and elevation gain, but if you are not acclimated to elevations above 5,000 feet, this hike will feel strenuous. Plan accordingly.

CONTACTS: 828-675-4611, ncparks.gov/mount-mitchell-state-park

Mount Mitchell High Loop

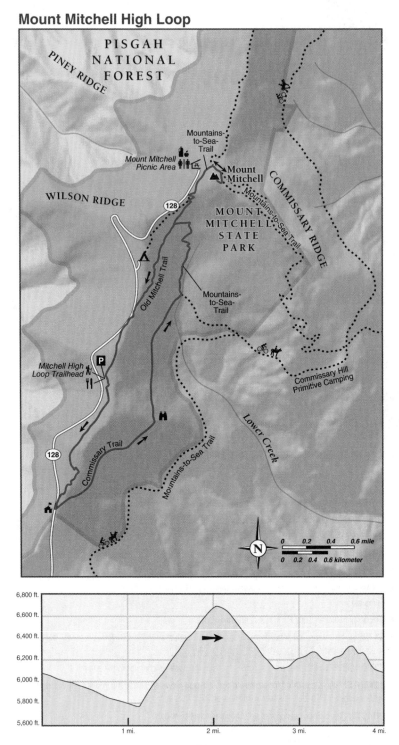

Overview

In 1835, professor, explorer, and scientist Elisha Mitchell measured this mountain—that in the future would be named after him—and proclaimed it to be the tallest summit between the Gulf of Mexico and the White Mountains of New Hampshire. This discovery brought researchers, commerce, and tourists to the Black Mountain Range. Today, we know that Mount Mitchell, at 6,684 feet, is the tallest mountain east of the Mississippi River. The Mount Mitchell High Loop first descends the historic Old Mitchell Trail; follows an old railroad bed to the top of the mountain, where Elisha Mitchell is buried; and finally returns to the trailhead through a dense Fraser fir forest.

Route Details

To begin the hike, park at the large lot where the park restaurant is located, then head south on the Old Mitchell Trail, rolling through spruce-fir forest with occasional openings where you can glimpse the mountains beyond. After 0.6 mile, you will come to the quaint state park office. Trail parking at the office is discouraged these days, but the rangers inside are friendly and helpful. Circle around the office and join the Commissary Trail, now northbound. The Commissary Trail follows an old railroad bed that was built at the turn of the 20th century. The railroad ran west to Pensacola, North Carolina, and south to Black Mountain, North Carolina. After two decades of logging, most of the Black Mountain slopes were barren.

In 1915, in an attempt to protect the remaining trees on top of Mount Mitchell, the North Carolina State Legislature designated the mountain and surrounding area as the first state park in North Carolina. Soon after, the logging train system converted to passenger rail that brought tourists to the top of the mountain. In 1922, the railroad bed was transformed into a toll road. The toll road remained the state park's main access road until the Mount Mitchell section of the Blue Ridge Parkway was built in 1939.

Today, the old toll road is lined with blueberry bushes, blackberry bushes, and stalks of goldenrod that attract butterflies in late summer. After you hike 1.2 miles, a view from the old toll road opens up; on a clear day you can see the summit of Mount Mitchell and Commissary Ridge skirting off to its right.

After completing 1.8 miles of your hike, you will reach a stream that runs across the gravel road. Just before the stream is a trail junction. Turn left and follow the combined Mountains-to-Sea Trail (MST) and Camp Alice Trail uphill into the dense forest. There, the heavy moss, dark canopy, and copious evergreens more closely resemble northern New England than the Southern Appalachians. And the ensuing shortness of breath reminds you that you are rising above 6,000 feet.

In 0.4 mile the Old Mitchell Trail intersects the MST. Continue uphill on the MST, but take special note of the yellow-blazed Old Mitchell Trail, as it will serve as your return route to the trailhead. Leaving the Old Mitchell Trail behind, you will switchback up the mountain several more times before passing the Campground Trail to the left. Stay with the MST, ascending the south slope of Mount Mitchell. In another 0.2 mile the dirt path terminates at the paved trail leading uphill 0.1 mile to the top of Mount Mitchell.

Congratulations! You have now climbed to the top of the tallest mountain in the eastern United States. Take a moment at the top to catch your breath and enjoy the view. You may also want to take a moment beneath the observation tower to visit the grave of Elisha Mitchell, an important figure in North Carolina history.

An ordained minister, Mitchell was also a professor at the University of North Carolina at Chapel Hill. The North Carolina Geological Survey brought him to the Black Mountain Range, and in 1835 he followed scientific protocol to measure and conclude that Mount Mitchell was the highest mountain between the Gulf of Mexico and Canada. However, in 1855, US Senator Thomas Clingman, a former student of Elisha Mitchell's, disputed his professor's claim. Clingman pronounced that Mitchell had mistakenly measured another peak along the Black Mountain Crest and named it as the tallest mountain. He suggested that he was the first to accurately measure the height of Mount Mitchell and confirm it as the tallest mountain in the East.

Here's what happened: Elisha Mitchell had returned to the Black Mountain Range in 1857 to validate his research, and he tragically lost his life at modern-day Mitchell Falls, when he slipped on a wet rock and tumbled to his death. Today, Elisha Mitchell and Thomas Clingman are both recognized as pioneers, and their legacies are remembered by respective 6,000-foot peaks named in their honor.

Leaving the summit, retrace your steps on the MST downhill through the forest to the junction with the Old Mitchell Trail. Turn south on the Old Mitchell

Trail and follow the yellow blazes painted on the trunks of sweet-smelling Fraser fir trees. The benefit of returning to the trailhead on the Old Mitchell Trail is that, after 0.8 mile, the path takes you back to the state park's restaurant, open during the warm season.

Nearby Attractions

Mount Mitchell has a restaurant, gift shop, and snack bar that are open to the public from May to October. The restaurant is 0.6 mile past the park office and is accessible by NC 128 or the Mount Mitchell High Loop. There is also a snack bar and gift shop at the end of NC 128.

Directions

Take the Blue Ridge Parkway north from Asheville. At mile marker 355, approximately 30 miles from Asheville, turn left onto NC 128. NC 128 leads into Mount Mitchell State Park. After 3.0 miles on NC 128, you will arrive at the Mount Mitchell State Park restaurant. Park there to begin the hike.

Mount Mitchell Circuit

SCENERY: ★ ★ ★ ★ ★
TRAIL CONDITION: ★ ★ ★
CHILDREN: ★
DIFFICULTY: ★ ★ ★ ★ ★
SOLITUDE: ★ ★

A HOST OF CAROLINA MOUNTAINS CAN BE SEEN FROM THE CREST OF BLACK MOUNTAIN.

TRAILHEAD GPS COORDINATES: 35.766200, -82.265317

DISTANCE & CONFIGURATION: 10.5-mile balloon

HIKING TIME: 8 hours

HIGHLIGHTS: The varied terrain and trails of Mount Mitchell State Park and the tallest mountain east of the Mississippi River

ELEVATION: 5,693' at Deep Gap. 6,684' on top of Mount Mitchell

ACCESS: Vehicle access may be limited in winter due to Blue Ridge Parkway closures. Check nps.gov/blri for real-time road closures.

MAPS: Mount Mitchell State Park; USGS *Mount Mitchell*

FACILITIES: Gift shop, snack bar, and restrooms at the trailhead parking area in season

WHEELCHAIR ACCESS: Yes, in the facilities, and also on a 0.2-mile trail to the Mount Mitchell summit

COMMENTS: Because weather can change very quickly above 6,000 feet, bring sunscreen, raingear, and warm clothes for layering.

CONTACTS: 828-675-4611, ncparks.gov/mount-mitchell-state-park

Overview

This hike is not direct, but it is adventurous. This route will not just take you to the top of Mount Mitchell; it will also explore neighboring summits on the Black Mountain Crest Trail before arriving at Deep Gap. From Deep Gap you will retrace your steps to the base of Big Tom Mountain before veering down to meet the Buncombe Horse Range Trail. Once on that trail, you will follow an old railroad bed that gently contours the mountain up to Commissary Ridge. One last uphill push on the Mountains-to-Sea Trail (MST) will lead to the 6,684-foot Mount Mitchell summit.

Route Details

It is worth reiterating that this route is an explorer circuit, designed to expose you to some of the most popular trails and different ecosystems within Mount Mitchell State Park. If you want a moderate and concise hike to the summit of Mount Mitchell, you may prefer the Mount Mitchell High Loop hike (see page 87). But if you want to take a full day exploring the Black Mountain Range, then this hike is for you.

The hike starts at the parking area below the Mount Mitchell summit, near the Mount Mitchell Gift Shop and Snack Bar. From the gift shop, follow the road east out of the main parking lot to reach the Mount Mitchell picnic area. This is the start of the Black Mountain Crest Trail. Follow the gravel path beside the picnic pavilion and between scattered picnic tables until it becomes a well-defined cut through the surrounding fir trees.

The Black Mountain Crest Trail will take you over some very prominent peaks on your hike to Deep Gap. The first summit you reach is Mount Craig. At 6,647 feet, Mount Craig is the second-highest mountain in the eastern United States. The peak is named for former North Carolina Governor Locke Craig, who established Mount Mitchell State Park as North Carolina's first state park and consequently helped protect the slopes of the Black Mountain Range from further logging.

From Mount Craig you will travel a short descent and then hike back uphill to reach the summit of Big Tom. Big Tom was named for Tom Wilson, a legendary mountaineer and bear hunter in the Black Mountain Range during the 1800s. Past Big Tom, you will once again descend into a neighboring gap,

Mount Mitchell Circuit

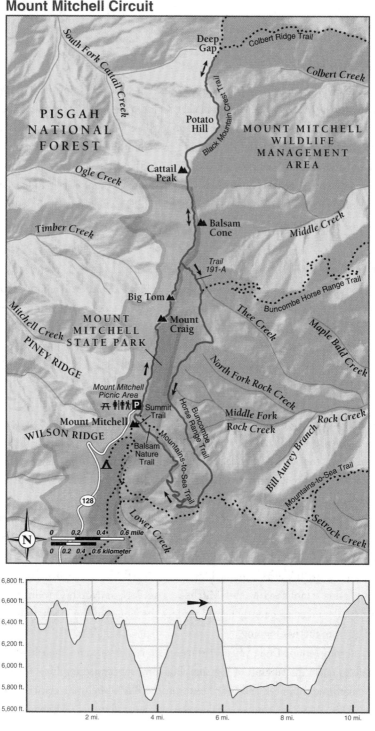

where Trail 191-A veers off to the east. If the first 1.7 miles of continuous up-and-down hiking has been more difficult than you expected, you may want to consider shaving off a total of 4 miles of undulating hills by turning east and shortcutting the loop. However, if you wish to continue on the Black Mountain Crest Trail to reach Deep Gap, then keep hiking north.

The next 2 miles leading to Deep Gap will take you through more of the dense spruce and fir forest that defines the ridgeline. This type of high-elevation evergreen forest is very rare in the southeastern United States; it exists only at the highest ridges of the Southern Appalachians, where the elevation and colder temperatures are too harsh for broadleaf hardwood trees to survive.

Continuing its up-and-down rhythm, the trail will take you over Balsam Cone, Cattail Peak, and Potato Hill before descending into Deep Gap. Deep Gap is unmarked, but it represents the northern boundary of Mount Mitchell State Park and has several backcountry campsites. Deep Gap is a good place to stop and enjoy a rest and bite of food before backtracking on the roller coaster of a ridge to Trail 191-A.

Once you retrace your steps along the crest to reach Trail 191-A at the base of Big Tom, turn east and follow the trail 0.5 mile downhill to meet Trail 191, the Buncombe Horse Range Trail. As a word of precaution, 191-A can become overgrown, especially during the summer months. Depending on the trail condition, you may have to bushwhack a little bit to reach the Buncombe Horse Range Trail. Be extra cautious to avoid plants with thorns on them, as this section is dotted with blackberry bushes, which might not be such a bad thing in late summer!

Past the weeds and bramble of 191-A, the Buncombe Horse Range Trail opens into a wide and level path that follows the old rail tramway that used to transport tourists to the top of Mount Mitchell. Your legs will appreciate this relatively flat 2.2-mile stretch, but be careful, as the trail does not have a good drainage system in place and can often become very muddy after a heavy rain.

After 8.7 miles of total hiking, you will come to an intersection with the MST. The MST coincides with the Buncombe Horse Range Trail for 200 yards, then veers northwest up Commissary Ridge. Follow the MST up the ridgeline. You will know you are getting closer to the Mount Mitchell summit when the MST joins the Balsam Nature Trail and informational placards appear on the side of the trail. At 10.3 miles the trail exits the woods and joins with a paved trail leading to the nearby Mount Mitchell Summit and Observation Tower. Take this trail to the summit and then follow it 0.2 mile downhill, past the MST, Balsam Nature Trail, Environmental Education Center, and Old Mitchell Trail, to complete your hike.

Nearby Attractions

Mount Mitchell's restaurant, gift shop, and snack bar are open to the public from May to October. The restaurant is 0.6 mile past the park office and is accessible by NC 128 or the Mount Mitchell High Loop (see page 87). There is also a snack bar and gift shop beneath the Mitchell summit at the end of NC 128.

Directions

Take the Blue Ridge Parkway north from Asheville. At mile marker 355, approximately 30 miles from Asheville, turn left onto NC 128. NC 128 leads into Mount Mitchell State Park. Drive 3 miles on NC 128 until it dead-ends at the Mount Mitchell Summit parking area.

THIS PICNIC SHELTER STANDS NEAR THE BEGINNING OF THE BLACK MOUNTAIN CREST TRAIL.

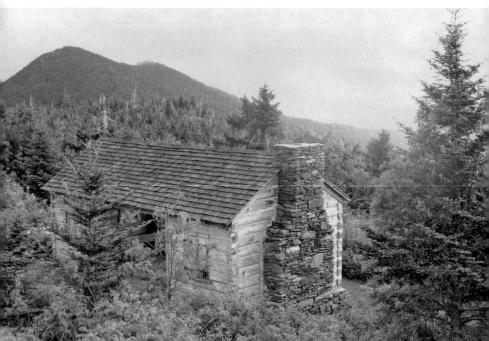

Setrock Creek Falls

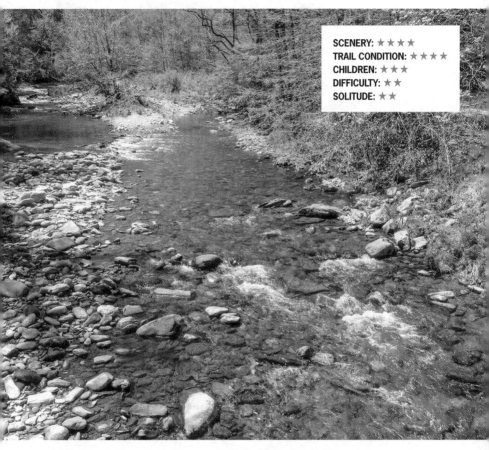

SCENERY: ★ ★ ★ ★
TRAIL CONDITION: ★ ★ ★ ★
CHILDREN: ★ ★ ★
DIFFICULTY: ★ ★
SOLITUDE: ★ ★

THIS HIKE MAKES A LOOP AROUND CRYSTALLINE SOUTH TOE RIVER.

TRAILHEAD GPS COORDINATES: 35.751001, -82.220036

DISTANCE & CONFIGURATION: 4.0-mile loop with spur to Setrock Creek Falls

HIKING TIME: 2.3 hours

HIGHLIGHTS: Setrock Creek Falls, South Toe River, Black Mountain Campground

ELEVATION: 3,000' at trailhead, 3,260' at high point

ACCESS: No fees or permits required

MAPS: National Geographic #779 *Pisgah National Forest: Linville Gorge Mount Mitchell*; USGS *Celo, Old Fort*

FACILITIES: Restroom at trailhead, full-service campground along hike, group campground

WHEELCHAIR ACCESS: One portion of trail near Black Mountain Campground

CONTACTS: Pisgah National Forest, 828-689-9694, fs.usda.gov/nfsnc

Setrock Creek Falls

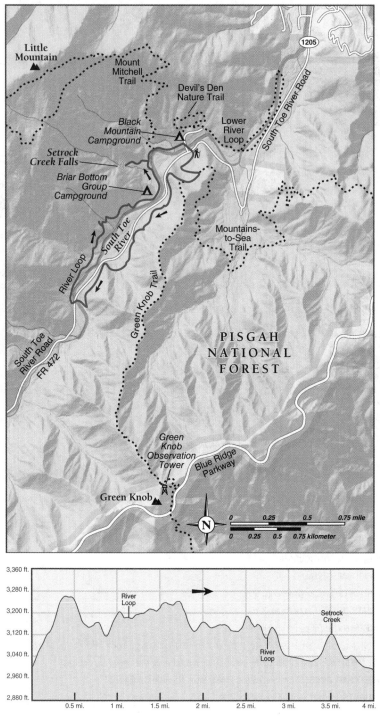

Overview

Enjoy a fun family trek, walking the hills and banks of the upper South Toe River, which drains the highlands of Mount Mitchell. Begin at the popular trailhead just outside of Pisgah National Forest's Black Mountain Campground, then weave your way to bridge the South Toe River, turning downstream. On the return, enjoy river views and then take the spur to 65-foot Setrock Creek Falls. Finally, cruise through Black Mountain Campground, checking out campsites for present or future camping trips that can expand your time here with swimming, tubing, fishing, or climbing to Mount Mitchell, in addition to this hike.

Route Details

The greater Black Mountain Recreation Area, part of the Pisgah National Forest in the shadow of hallowed Mount Mitchell, is the setting for this fine circuit hike that will leave you desiring some aquatic mountain fun. Best enjoyed from late spring through late summer, this easy to moderate loop explores the South Toe River and one of its tributaries—Setrock Creek, where the stream falls in stages down, down, down, widening before the cataract expires in a shallow splash pool. The waterfall is a popular quick destination for those overnighting at Black Mountain Campground, a recommended facility with reservable sites that you should incorporate into a trip here. In addition to water activities, avid Asheville hikers can use the Black Mountain trailhead to make the challenging climb to Mount Mitchell, do the lower River Loop, trek a portion of the Mountains-to-Sea Trail, or jaunt down the Devils Den Nature Trail.

There's a lot to do here, and the big trailhead parking area evinces it. From the trailhead kiosk, begin your clockwise circuit on the River Loop, sharing the path with the Green Knob Trail and the Mountains-to-Sea Trail. Though the loop has significant few climbs, the first part of the hike delivers the primary ascent—270 feet in the first 0.4 mile, where you part ways with the Mountains-to-Sea Trail at 0.3 mile, then with the Green Knob Trail at 0.4 mile. (Aggregate elevation gain/loss on the entire hike is 744 feet.) From there, the path is less rocky as you head south with the South Toe River, stepping over feeder branches spilling toward the South Toe. Listen for river sounds below as you ramble along the lower slope of Lost Cove Ridge.

At 1.6 miles, come near gravel South Toe River Road, FR 472, linking Black Mountain Recreation Area to the Blue Ridge Parkway. At 1.9 miles, reach FR 472 and use the road span to cross the South Toe River. Watch carefully for the River Loop trail blazes as they cut through a dispersed campsite. (Primitive, free campsites marked with brown tent symbol signs are situated upriver along FR 472 between this point and the Blue Ridge Parkway.) Stay with the blazes as you now turn downstream among brushy evergreens.

Although you are going downstream, the balance of the walk from here includes a little up to go along with the mostly down. Make a modest uptick after crossing Camp Creek at 2.4 miles, flowing off the slopes of Commissary Hill on the shoulder of Mount Mitchell. After working around Whiteside Ridge,

SPRING SURROUNDS SETROCK CREEK FALLS.

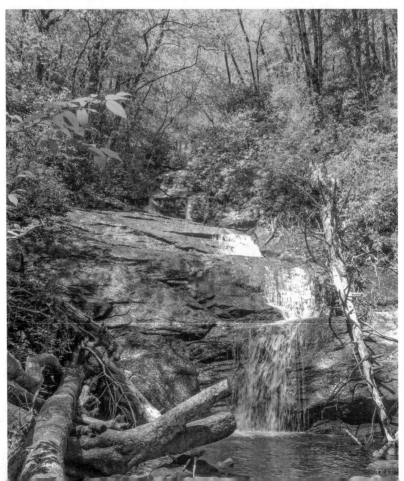

cross a smaller, cascade-rich stream. These cascades are more noticeable from winter through spring, or when the watercourse is running high.

At 3.0 miles, the River Loop takes you alongside the South Toe River, then into Briar Bottom Group Camp. Facilities may be closed if the camp is not being used. Continue down the trail beyond the camp, crossing campground access roads and staying with the River Loop blazes, then bridge Setrock Creek at 3.4 miles. At 3.5 miles, turn left on the Setrock Creek Falls Trail. The path shortly crosses another campground access road, and it is but 0.1 mile to the base of the 65-foot welter of whitewater. Like other small watershed cataracts, Setrock Creek Falls flows are seasonal. In winter and spring, the cataract will crash brash and defiant, lessening through the summer until it can be a murmuring disappointment during a dry autumn. After backtracking to the River Loop, cross a metal span over another stream. Watch for spur trails linking to the Briar Bottom access road.

At 3.8 miles, the Mount Mitchell Trail leaves left and climbs 3,600+ challenging feet to the top of Mount Mitchell. The River Loop keeps straight and continues parallel to the South Toe River, elevated in places, delivering a top-down look at the crystalline stream, separated from the path by a wooden fence in places. At 4.0 miles, pop out near the Black Mountain Campground office to turn right and cross an auto bridge before reaching the trailhead where the River Loop began.

Nearby Attractions

Black Mountain Recreation offers 37 widespread campsites set in a pretty flat along the South Toe River. Open seasonally. Visit recreation.gov for more information.

Directions

From Asheville, take the Blue Ridge Parkway north for 31 miles. Turn left onto gravel South Toe River Road, FR 472, and descend for 4.5 miles to reach the Black Mountain trailhead on the right, at the bridge leaving left into the Black Mountain Campground.

Snooks Nose
and Hickory Branch Falls

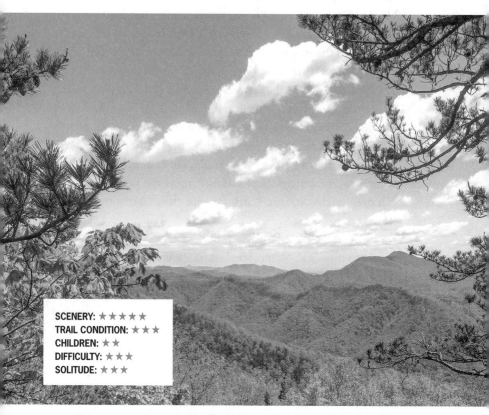

SCENERY: ★ ★ ★ ★ ★
TRAIL CONDITION: ★ ★ ★
CHILDREN: ★ ★
DIFFICULTY: ★ ★ ★
SOLITUDE: ★ ★ ★

SCANNING NORTHEAST ACROSS CURTIS CREEK TO MACKEY MOUNTAIN AND BEYOND

TRAILHEAD GPS COORDINATES: 35.690850, -82.196467

DISTANCE & CONFIGURATION: 4.4- and 1.2-mile out-and-backs

HIKING TIME: 2.9 hours for both hikes

HIGHLIGHTS: Views from Snooks Nose, Hickory Branch Falls, Slick Falls

ELEVATION: 1,880' at trailhead, 3,680' on Snooks Nose

ACCESS: Free and always open

MAPS: National Geographic #779 *Pisgah National Forest: Linville Gorge Mount Mitchell;* USGS *Old Fort*

FACILITIES: Campground, picnic area at trailhead

WHEELCHAIR ACCESS: None

CONTACTS: Pisgah National Forest, Grandfather Ranger District, 828-652-2144, fs.usda.gov/nfsnc

Overview

This adventure features two fun yet dissimilar hikes from the same trailhead. Take the steep Snooks Nose Trail past Slick Falls up to outcrops on Snooks Nose, presenting rewarding east and west panoramas of the Blue Ridge and adjacent mountains. Cap off this first hike with an easy walk to attractive Hickory Branch Falls, a 20-foot tumbling froth of white. Furthermore, you can picnic or camp at the trailhead, since the two hikes begin at the Pisgah National Forest's Curtis Creek Campground.

Route Details

Who wouldn't want to hike to a destination known as Snooks Nose? Though it is only 2.2 miles to the rewarding views from Snooks Nose, the climb is a whopping 1,800 feet over those 2 miles! Your second adventure is a 0.6-mile one-way walk to Hickory Branch Falls, where the climb is a mere 220 feet. Hickory Branch tumbles through a deep vale hemmed in by Buckeye Knob and Moses Ridge. During its frothy flow through crowded rhododendron thickets and rising hardwoods, Hickory Branch finds an erosion-resistant cliff, spilling into a gravelly pool ensconced in vegetation. You can do one hike or the other, or both. It is super convenient being able to accomplish both treks from the same trailhead.

Finding the Snooks Nose Trail can be problematic. From the picnic area parking, backtrack on foot down Curtis Creek Road, crossing Curtis Creek on the road bridge. Continue south and after 0.1 mile, the signed singletrack Snooks Nose Trail leaves right, across the road from Campsite 10.

Notorious for its steep sections, you are expecting the Snooks Nose Trail to ascend immediately, but it doesn't, instead tracing an old forest road around a ridge before turning into Slick Falls Branch watershed. The richly wooded vale narrows. At 0.5 mile, rock-hop placid Slick Falls Branch. The ascent finally begins. At 0.8 mile, a short, steep spur trail drops right to Slick Falls Branch. The actual Slick Falls is a little upstream of the water access, blocked by a compact rhododendron thicket. To climb directly up the watercourse is folly (they don't call it Slick Falls for nothing); therefore, exercise extreme caution trying to visit this 100-plus-foot spiller.

Snooks Nose and Hickory Branch Falls

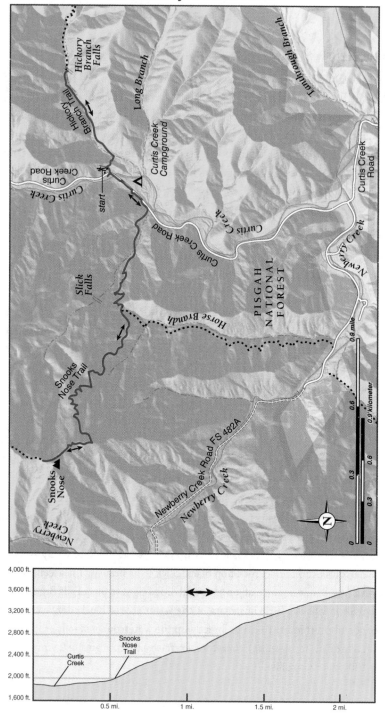

At 0.9 mile, the Snooks Nose Trail briefly levels in a gap. Here, an unnamed old forest road descends straight, heading along Horse Branch about 1.2 miles down to Newberry Creek Road. Your hike splits right, westerly, angling up a slope toward Snooks Nose, still on the Snooks Nose Trail. Work through some of the infamous steep sections while amidst mountain laurel thickets. Note the blackened trunks of trees and brush from past prescribed burns. Switchbacks ease the climb, and at 1.9 miles you turn north onto the tip of Snooks Nose. Continue your upward tick, tickling Snooks Nose, and at 2.1 miles, level out atop a narrow, rocky ridgeline dotted with scrubby pines and other brushy vegetation. Fine vistas open to your west and east. The Blue Ridge and the Craggies stand across the Newberry Creek to west. To the east and northeast rise forested mounts and stream-laden valleys of the Pisgah National Forest, most notably Curtis Creek, from which you rose. Relax, pull up a rock, and savor the panoramas. From here, the Snooks Nose Trail continues about 2 miles to Green Knob and the Blue Ridge Parkway.

Consider adding the short family walk to Hickory Branch Falls, starting from the same parking area as Snooks Nose. Find campsite 21 across from the Curtis Creek picnic area parking, then make a little climb over a hill down to the valley of Hickory Branch, quickly traversing the stream. This crossing will alert you to whether or not the falls will be flowing boldly. Continue on the right bank, heading upstream amidst evergreens aplenty. Cross back over to the left bank of Hickory Branch at 0.3 mile. The streamside flat ends and the valley sharpens, setting the stage for a mountain cataract. Hickory Branch tumbles louder ahead. Step over a small tributary flowing down the hollow to your left, then come to Hickory Branch Falls at 0.6 mile, making its 20-foot slide over a rock face. You can photograph it from the trail or at its base. From here, the Hickory Branch Trail climbs out of its watershed to meet the Lead Mine Gap Trail on Chestnutwood Mountain. After viewing the falls, perhaps enhance your adventure with a picnic or campout at Curtis Creek Campground.

Nearby Attractions

You'll pass through the quaint town of Old Fort en route to the hike. Its downtown is worth a little exploration.

Directions

From Exit 72 on I-40 east of Asheville, take Main Street/US 70 east through Old Fort. At 2.6 miles, turn left on Curtis Creek Road. Follow the paved road as it turns to gravel and reaches a gate at 4.6 miles. You will have to park here when the campground is closed (usually from January 1 through March 31); otherwise, proceed up the forest road for 0.6 mile farther to reach the campground after a total of 5.2 miles. Bridge Curtis Creek, then park in the creekside spots on the left near the upper part of the campground, above the paved campground loop.

HICKORY BRANCH FALLS

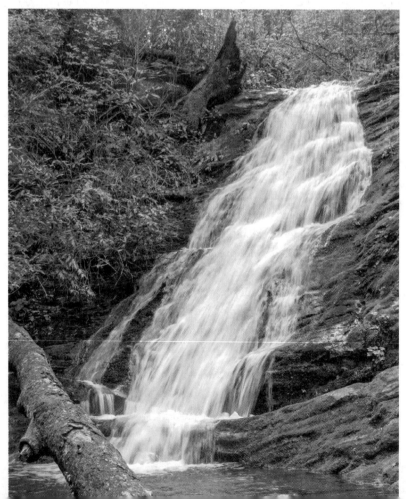

Bearwallow Mountain

LOOKING SOUTH FROM BEARWALLOW MOUNTAIN

TRAILHEAD GPS COORDINATES: 35.460650, -82.367867

DISTANCE & CONFIGURATION: 2-mile out-and-back or loop

HIKING TIME: 1.5 hours

HIGHLIGHTS: Distant panoramas from mountaintop meadow

ELEVATION: 3,640' at trailhead, 4,232' at highest point

ACCESS: No fees or permits required

MAPS: Bearwallow Mountain Trail; USGS *Bat Cave*

FACILITIES: None

WHEELCHAIR ACCESS: None

CONTACTS: Carolina Mountain Land Conservancy, 828-697-5777, carolinamountain.org

Bearwallow Mountain

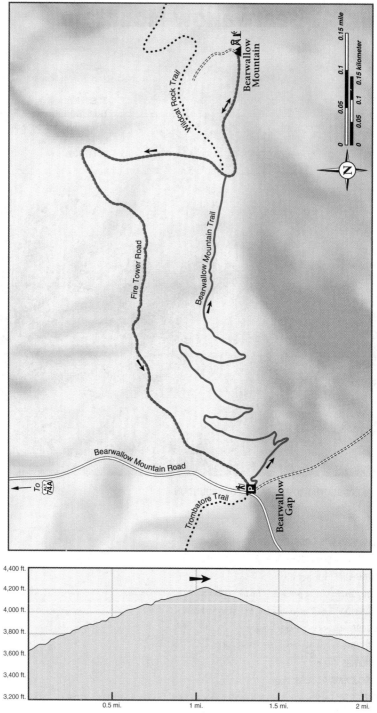

Overview

Home to breathtaking vistas and at least seven rare plant species, this preserve
is managed by the Carolina Mountain Land Conservancy (CMLC) and features
a fine wildflower-rich trail leading up to a grassy bald and its preeminent views.
A historic fire tower (currently closed) complements the scene. This is one peak
nearly everyone can bag because the hike is short and fairly easy.

Back in 1934, at a time when only cows were enjoying the views from
the meadows of Bearwallow Mountain, the Civilian Conservation Corps built
a fire tower from which rangers could monitor the skies from the lookout atop
the 47-foot steel structure. The tower was in use for six decades, primarily
during the spring and fall fire seasons, though earlier stints lasted continuously
from December through April. During that time a ranger would stay in a rough
on-site cabin, later to be replaced by a wood-frame house.

During that period, a road ran to the tower site. As time went on and
word of the views spread, curious locals would park at Bearwallow Gap and
walk up the road to experience what the rangers enjoyed atop the tower, such
as sights of downtown Asheville, Lake Lure, the Black Mountains, Hickorynut
Gorge, and even the crags of Great Smoky Mountains National Park. Although
the surreptitious visitors couldn't climb the tower, the views were still stunning.
Eventually, the tower was decommissioned and closed, though it still stands. In
the future, the tower may be restored and open to the public. Nevertheless, the
panoramas from atop Bearwallow Mountain will more than sate the appetite of
any view-hungry peak bagger.

Bearwallow Mountain became one of those cool, undercover hiking destinations for Ashevillians. The only problem was that hiking there wasn't quite
legal. In stepped the CMLC. It bought an 81-acre conservation easement atop
Bearwallow Mountain, then built a hiking trail to the top. And now we can hike
it without compunction. You have the option of turning your hike into a loop
by taking the old fire road used by Bearwallow Mountain rangers and visitors
from days gone by. The conservancy has since added 84 more easement acres on
Bearwallow Mountain.

Route Details

Save this hike for a clear day and you will be well rewarded. By the way, it is a
good starter "mountain climb" for younger hikers. When leaving Bearwallow

Gap for the hike, be sure to join the Bearwallow Mountain Trail, rather than the Trombatore Trail across the road (although that is a worthwhile endeavor). The Bearwallow Mountain Trail leaves east from the gap, along with the old road access to Bearwallow Mountain. The footpath makes a series of switchbacks under a mantle of buckeye trees, along with oaks and hickories. Trilliums bloom by the score along the slopes in spring. Note the extensive trail work done by the CMLC with the wood-and-earth stairs that ease the ascent and prevent erosion.

After a half mile, the Bearwallow Mountain Trail crosses the top of a bluff. Trees are already becoming more stunted by the elevation and exposure on the upward slopes. At 0.7 mile the path slips alongside a boulder garden, amid stones large and small. Ahead, you may notice more light. And at 0.8 mile

THE OLD FIRE WATCHERS' TOWER

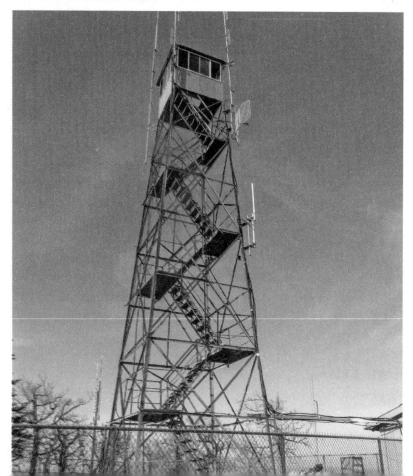

the trail emerges onto the grassy slopes of Bearwallow Mountain. You will notice that Bearwallow now contains more than a decommissioned fire tower and ranger house. The peak is dotted with communication towers for uses from smartphones to county emergency services.

At this point you may feel like roaming the bald. However, a bit ahead is the access road to the top. I suggest bagging the peak and checking out the fire tower and facilities at the top. It's less than a quarter mile away. Once atop the bald, explore as you please. Check out the grassy meadows occasionally poked with rocks. Wind-shaped trees border the edges of the field. Additionally, the 5.0-mile Wildcat Rock Trail leads past a view and down to US 74A.

Look northwest for the buildings of downtown Asheville. This is where a pair of binoculars comes in handy. You can make out specific buildings—and perhaps see your jealous friends stuck in the office while you scan for more highland panoramas. The ridgeline of the Black Mountain Range is to the north, while a host of mountains stretches to the south. Thank the CMLC while lauding these vistas.

Finally, you can return via the trail, backtracking, or walk the mountain road to create a loop. The road is easier on the feet. Today, the track is primarily used by those attending the many towers atop Bearwallow Mountain, while the trail is left to us hikers.

Nearby Attractions

The Trombatore Trail also starts at Bearwallow Gap and leads 2.5 miles one way to a vista from Blue Ridge Pastures. Expect the trail system in this area to expand under the guidance of the CMLC.

Directions

From downtown Asheville, take I-240 east to Exit 9, Blue Ridge Parkway/Bat Cave, joining US 74A. Take US 74A east for 12.7 miles to turn right on Bearwallow Mountain Road, a little before the Gerton post office. Trace Bearwallow Mountain Road for 2.1 miles to Bearwallow Gap. Be very careful and park only in allowed spots. Don't block the road.

19 Florence Nature Preserve

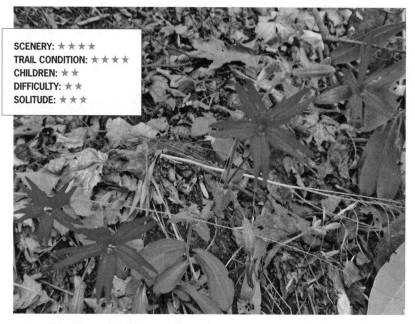

SCENERY: ★ ★ ★ ★
TRAIL CONDITION: ★ ★ ★ ★
CHILDREN: ★ ★
DIFFICULTY: ★ ★
SOLITUDE: ★ ★ ★

FIRE PINKS LINE THE TRAIL.

TRAILHEAD GPS COORDINATES: 35.473350, -82.332117
DISTANCE & CONFIGURATION: 5.3-mile balloon
HIKING TIME: 3.2 hours
HIGHLIGHTS: Waterfalls, views, wildflowers
ELEVATION: 2,460' at trailhead, 3,360' at highest point
ACCESS: No fees or permits required
MAPS: Florence Nature Preserve; USGS *Bat Cave*
FACILITIES: None
WHEELCHAIR ACCESS: None
CONTACTS: Carolina Mountain Land Conservancy, 828-697-5777, carolinamountain.org

Overview

A hike through this private preserve managed by the Carolina Mountain Land Conservancy (CMLC) displays a selection of Southern Appalachian splendor as it loops along the Blue Ridge. Start with a climb along the slopes of Burntshirt Mountain (on the all-time best North Carolina place name list), and then circle through the preserve, once the retreat of a retired Atlanta doctor. While coursing through this outpost you will find wildflowers galore, so stop for a view. Wander amid regal and varied woodlands. Stop at a second outcrop and soak in another vista. The final part of the loop climbs a stream, where a pair of dissimilar cataracts provides a double dose of aquatic excitement.

The transformation that lands in Western North Carolina have undergone over the past century is amazing. And the Florence Nature Preserve tract exemplifies those changes. More than a century ago, this land was home to several subsistence farms, where backwoods families lived a simple life, growing and providing most items needed for their existence, save for items such as coffee. These people lived quiet lives hoeing corn on hillsides; maybe growing tobacco to pay their land taxes; running a pig or two through the woods; and, if they were lucky, having a milk cow. However, the sloped terrain was susceptible to erosion and the land grew less fertile. Decreased productivity and mill jobs eventually lured theses farmers off the land. The forest grew back, and Carolina's mountains became a scenic retreat for men like Dr. Tom Florence, an Atlanta doctor who, back in 1966, bought 600 acres in these majestic highlands. After enjoying his retreat for decades, the next step would be to sell the land for a gated mountain community. However, Dr. Florence donated his enclave to the CMLC, desiring to keep the land in a natural state. The conservancy has since created a system of color-coded trails, traversing the tract's highlights.

Route Details

This hike leaves the trailhead, once a mountainside cabin homesite, and ascends a narrow, yellow-blazed path, winding the north slope of Burntshirt Mountain. At 0.3 mile come to a trailside spring. At 0.4 mile use an intriguing stone slab bridge to span a streamlet. The path winds around a hollow, then comes to a tributary of Hickory Creek at 0.8 mile. Ascend the right bank of the stream before crossing it at 0.9 mile, and reach a trail intersection.

Begin the loop, heading counterclockwise, northbound on the slopes of Little Pisgah Mountain, joining the Blue Trail as it ascends the rhododendron-canopied stream. At 1.2 miles you will reach the cabin site of one of the aforementioned hardscrabble farms. Look for the stone foundation and chimney. Consider the lives led here, the people who sat before the chimney hearth. At

Florence Nature Preserve

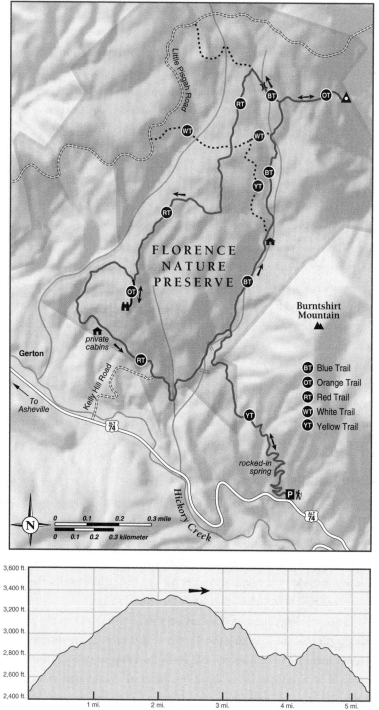

Burntshirt Mountain

BT Blue Trail
OT Orange Trail
RT Red Trail
WT White Trail
YT Yellow Trail

Gerton

To Asheville

private cabins

Little Pisgah Road

Kelly Hill Road

FLORENCE NATURE PRESERVE

rocked-in spring

Hickory Creek

ALT 74

N

0   0.1   0.2   0.3 mile
0   0.1   0.2   0.3 kilometer

1.3 miles the Yellow Trail heads left. Keep straight on the Blue Trail and pass the intersection with the White Trail at 1.5 miles.

Ready to grab a view? At 1.7 miles turn right on the Orange Trail and reach a rock crag at 1.9 miles, where you can look east toward the Carolina Piedmont. The views are better in leafless winter. Backtrack, then rejoin the Blue Trail. Turn left on the Red Trail after crossing a creek on a seemingly out-of-place

THE VIEW ACROSS THE HICKORY CREEK VALLEY

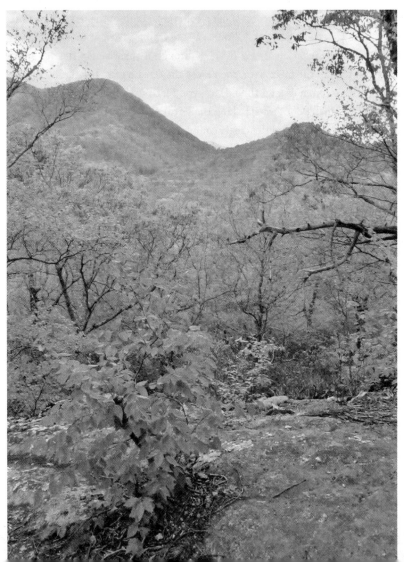

road bridge. Bisect the White Trail at 2.5 miles, heading south, away from Little Pisgah Mountain.

Ready for another view? At 3.1 miles meet the Orange Trail and climb a hill 0.1 mile to an outcrop where the far side of the Hickory Creek valley rises. Backtrack and rejoin the Red Trail. The path descends sharply. At 3.6 miles the trail turns sharply left, where you join an old roadbed. At 3.7 miles, the trail winds past private cabins, where the route follows the gravel cabin access road, an extension of Kelly Hill Road.

At 4 miles the path heads left as a narrow trail where Kelly Hill Road leaves right. Soon you'll cross a small creek, then climb to the next creek over, where the waterfalls flow. At 4.2 miles a side trail leads right to a fascinating waterfall. This spiller slides for 60 feet through a surprisingly slender stone chute. Return to the main path, then cross the stream of the waterfall. Ahead, bridge the stream a second time. Here, you reach a 15-foot, two-tier cataract ending in a small pool. Ascend along the left bank of the stream. Beyond this second spiller, you ascend the creek, completing the loop portion of the hike at 4.4 miles. From here it is a 0.9-mile backtrack to the trailhead.

Nearby Attractions

The CMLC maintains other trails nearby, on the other side of the Hickory Creek valley. The Wildcat Rock starts its 5-mile journey just across the road from this hike. Bearwallow Mountain Trail leads 1 mile to a highland meadow and is detailed in this guide (see page 107). The Trombatore Trail also starts at Bearwallow Gap and leads 2.5 miles one way to a vista from Blue Ridge Pastures.

Directions

From downtown Asheville, take I-240 east to Exit 9, Blue Ridge Parkway/Bat Cave, joining US 74A. Take US 74A east 13.8 miles to the trailhead parking area on your left, 0.9 mile past the Upper Hickory Nut Gorge Community Center. Spaces are limited.

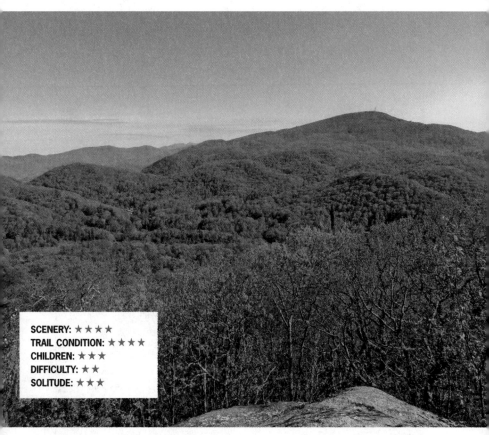

SCENERY: ★ ★ ★ ★
TRAIL CONDITION: ★ ★ ★ ★
CHILDREN: ★ ★ ★
DIFFICULTY: ★ ★
SOLITUDE: ★ ★ ★

WILDCAT ROCK FEATURES THIS LOOK NORTH AT 4,412-FOOT LITTLE PISGAH MOUNTAIN.

TRAILHEAD GPS COORDINATES: 35.473210, -82.331996

DISTANCE & CONFIGURATION: 3.2-mile out-and-back

HIKING TIME: 1.8 hours

HIGHLIGHTS: Views from Wildcat Rock, Little Bearwallow Falls

ELEVATION: 2,439' at trailhead, 3,415' at Bear Rock

ACCESS: No fees or permits required

MAPS: Upper Hickory Nut Gorge Trail System; USGS *Bat Cave*

FACILITIES: None

WHEELCHAIR ACCESS: None

CONTACTS: Conserving Carolina, 828-697-5777, conservingcarolina.org

Wildcat Rock

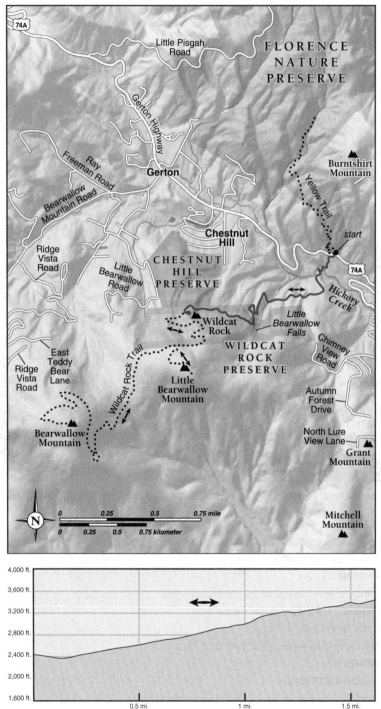

Overview

Take a hike on one of greater Asheville's newer trails. Start in the Upper Hickory Nut Gorge, climbing the north slope of Little Bearwallow Mountain after bridging Hickory Creek. Angle past Little Bearwallow Falls, spilling over a naked slab of stone. Skirt past more stone slopes before making a final climb to Wildcat Rock, where you find extensive views of the upper Hickory Creek valley backed by Little Pisgah Mountain, among other wooded peaks.

Route Details

The Upper Hickory Nut Gorge trail system continues to expand, thanks to the efforts of an outfit known as Conserving Carolina. Their mission is "to protect, restore, and inspire appreciation of the natural world." This includes purchasing and preserving highland destinations like Little Bearwallow Mountain (which we will explore on this hike), as well as streams, rivers, farms and more. Located on the south side of the Hickory Nut Gorge, with access at the exact trailhead for another Conserving Carolina success story—Florence Nature Preserve—the Wildcat Rock Trail takes you first through a private property easement (thanks, Laughing Waters retreat); down to burbling Hickory Creek, a cool, clear mountain stream; then up along a north-facing slope where wildflowers from trillium to jack-in-the-pulpit to Solomon's seal rise in profusion. A stop at Little Bearwallow Falls (best seen in winter as a frozen ice-climbing area or in spring with some decent flow) leads next to Wildcat Rock, where stunted trees border a north- and west-facing overlook that makes an ample reward for most hikers. If you desire, a little more climbing will take you to the open upper slopes of Little Bearwallow Mountain. *Note:* Please stay off signed private trails linking to the Wildcat Rock Trail.

When arriving at the trailhead, it's tempting to head north on the more obvious paths of Florence Nature Preserve (see page 112). Instead, look south across from the road from the parking area, finding a kiosk and the Wildcat Rock Trail. The Wildcat Rock Trail descends to run along a small orchard, part of Laughing Waters retreat, aiming for Hickory Creek at the base of the valley. Little Bearwallow Mountain rises across the vale. Look for open stone faces on the mountainside, below which you will walk later.

At 0.1 mile, the track enters woods. Crystalline Hickory Creek sings in your ears. Rhododendron and doghobble rise in thickets under black birches. Bridge a braid of Hickory Creek, then span Hickory Creek itself. The path circles downstream creekside before angling up the north slope of Little Bearwallow Mountain in its quest for Wildcat Rock and beyond. It is on this moist north-facing mountainside where wildflowers thrive. A well-timed April trip will deliver a cornucopia of color from these harbingers of spring, namely trilliums.

As you climb, note the first-rate stone, rock, and log work that went into building the trail, especially the steps you use to ascend. Sometimes, while hiking, I'll start flagging, but then I only need to consider the amount of energy used to construct the path itself, rather than merely hiking it, and am thus inspired. Hickory and oak increase in number as you ascend. At 0.7 mile step over the unnamed stream of Little Bearwallow Falls. Next, you rise near a boulder garden before reaching the base of Little Bearwallow Falls at 1.1 miles. Here, the seasonal stream leaves the woods and ventures onto a naked rock slab, sliding

SPRINGTIME WILL REVEAL TRILLIUMS EN ROUTE TO WILDCAT ROCK.

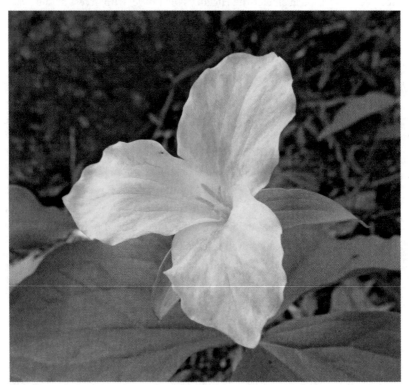

about 120 feet, then flowing past the trail. However, the small watershed of the stream leaves this cataract a dramatic sight only after heavy rains. Alas, it may dry up entirely in late summer and autumn. During winter, the watercourse often freezes and is used as an ice-climbing venue. Rock climbers also ply the open stone face throughout warmer times.

From there, the Wildcat Rock Trail climbs stone steps and then works west along the base of several rock slabs, some clothed in mosses, some with water dribbling over them. At 1.4 miles pass a small rock shelter. At 1.5 miles come to a trail intersection. Here, the now lesser-used Wildcat Rock Trail keeps straight while you split left on the spur to Wildcat Rock, twisting upward alongside a stone outcrop, trimmed in mountain laurel and small trees. Rise farther, then emerge onto Wildcat Rock, which is not that big but large enough to allow unimpeded vistas of the Hickory Creek Valley below and the crest of the Blue Ridge to your west and north, highlighted by 4,412-foot Little Pisgah Mountain and its telltale tower, with other peaks in the distance.

The Wildcat Rock trailbed shows most hikers trek to Wildcat Rock and its views, going no farther. However, more high-quality hiking on the Wildcat Rock Trail leads to the open slopes of Little Bearwallow Mountain and to the open, view-laden crest of Bearwallow Mountain itself. (For an alternative hike to Bearwallow Mountain from Bearwallow Gap, see page 107.) From Wildcat Rock it is 1.0 mile to the top of Little Bearwallow Mountain and 1.7 more miles to the top of Bearwallow Mountain.

Nearby Attractions

You can access the trails of Florence Nature Preserve from this same trailhead (see page 112).

Directions

From downtown Asheville, take I-240 east to Exit 9, Blue Ridge Parkway/Bat Cave, joining US 74A. Take US 74A east 13.8 miles to the trailhead parking area on your left, 0.9 mile past the Upper Hickory Nut Gorge Community Center. The Wildcat Rock Trail begins on the south side of US 74A.

South

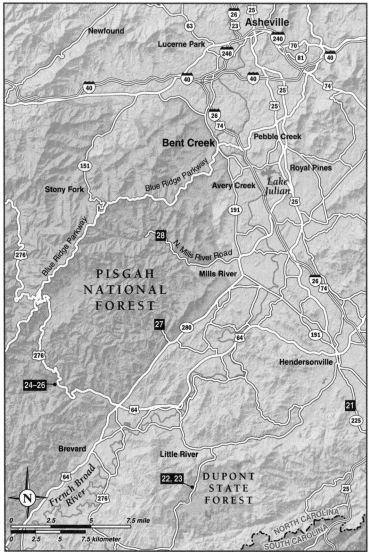

South

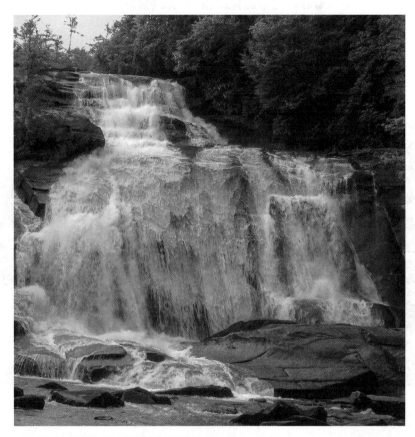

HIGH FALLS MAKES ITS POWERFUL CHARGE *(Hike 22, page 129)*.

21

Carl Sandburg's Connemara Farms

SCENERY: ★ ★ ★ ★
TRAIL CONDITION: ★ ★ ★ ★ ★
CHILDREN: ★ ★ ★ ★ ★
DIFFICULTY: ★ ★
SOLITUDE: ★

WITH VIEWS LIKE THIS, YOU CAN SEE WHY CARL SANDBURG CHOSE TO MAKE THIS SPOT HOME.

TRAILHEAD GPS COORDINATES: 35.273431, -82.444795

DISTANCE & CONFIGURATION: 4-mile out-and-back

HIKING TIME: 2.5 hours

HIGHLIGHTS: Carl Sandburg's homestead and great views from Glassy Mountain

ELEVATION: 2,163' at trailhead, 2,780' on Glassy Summit

ACCESS: The trailhead access is open year-round, sunrise–sunset; visitor center is open Thursday–Sunday from 10 a.m. to 4 p.m. There is no fee to access the grounds, hike the trails, or visit the dairy barn.

MAPS: USGS *Hendersonville*

FACILITIES: Restrooms at the bottom of the wheelchair ramp near the parking lot

WHEELCHAIR ACCESS: A shuttle is available from the parking lot kiosk to the Sandburg house.

COMMENTS: Fee-based guided tours of the Sandburg house are offered on weekends year-round. Reservations can be made through recreation.gov.

CONTACTS: 828-693-4178, nps.gov/carl

Overview

Showcasing Carl Sandburg's homestead, this route leads around the lake at the property's entrance, continues beside the white clapboard farmhouse, and heads up the hill for views from the exposed granite rock face on top of Glassy Mountain.

Route Details

The Pulitzer Prize–winning author and poet Carl Sandburg (1878–1967) retreated from Michigan to the mountains of North Carolina in 1945 to find seclusion and inspiration for his writing, as well as a more temperate climate for his wife's award-winning herd of dairy goats. At his home in Flat Rock, the writer spent 22 happy years in active retirement. In 1967, the Poet of the People passed away, and a year later the U.S. Congress designated Connemara, the family farm, as a National Historic Site. Today, the 264-acre country landscape is open to the public and offers 5 miles of well-maintained hiking trails.

The trail to the top of Glassy Mountain, the highest point on Connemara Farms, starts with a gentle warm-up loop around the 0.4-mile Lake Trail. To begin your hike, walk down the wheelchair ramp from the parking lot to the lake. Turn left and hike south on a dirt path that travels clockwise around the water.

After 0.2 mile the lake trail intersects a path leading to the Sandburg house. Stay on the Lake Trail and continue to hug the shoreline for 0.4 mile, until you reach a rock wall on your left. At the rock wall, turn left and walk uphill on a shaded dirt path that separates a grassy field on the left from a paved driveway on the right.

At the top of the hill, this 0.3-mile trail will terminate at a road intersection. To the left, the road leads to the Sandburg house and visitor center, but the hike continues straight and follows the road past the modern restroom facility and historic Connemara outbuildings. Just beyond the springhouse, the road turns right toward the goat barn. At this point the trail turns left and heads south beside the woodshed on a gentle uphill slope.

Hike steadily up the slight incline through a tunnel of mountain laurel bushes that typically show their pink-and-white blossoms in mid-May. A side trail to the left leads to views on top of Little Glassy Mountain, but by staying on the main path you will arrive at a four-way trail intersection after 0.9 mile of total walking.

Carl Sandburg's Connemara Farms

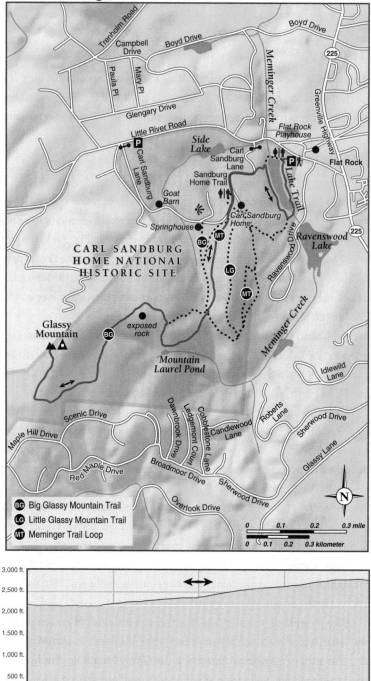

Big Glassy Mountain Trail

Little Glassy Mountain Trail

Meminger Trail Loop

At the intersection, do not turn to the left or right, but continue your hike on the Big Glassy Mountain Trail. You will know you are on the right trail when the grade of the path increases as it continues up the mountain. For 0.75 mile the trail ascends through a mixed forest of pine trees, tulip poplars, oak trees, and red maples. The heart-pounding climb is kindly broken into sections by wooden benches strategically placed on the side of the trail. Take time to sit by the small pond to the left of the trail, or stop at the next clearing to enjoy the yellow ragwort wildflowers (in spring) or watch a small lizard scurry across the gray granite rock.

After a cumulative 1.7 miles, the trail turns right and levels out along the ridge. Follow the path another 0.2 mile through the forest and across an exposed rock to reach a set of stairs that leads out to Glassy Mountain Overlook. The view from Glassy Mountain extends out over Etowah Valley and toward Mount Pisgah. With your eyes, follow the ridgeline from the tower on top of Mount Pisgah to the left and you will visually be able to trace the southwest route of the Blue Ridge Parkway.

After resting and enjoying the view on top of Glassy Mountain, return to the parking lot on the same route that took you there. Be sure to take a cool-down lap around the level lake trail to conclude the hike.

However, don't leave the property without visiting the dairy goats at the Goat Barn. The goats are a favorite with children and adults. These year-round residents are descendants of the prize-winning dairy goats that Carl Sandburg and his wife, Lilian, raised. The friendly animals roam free in an open field. In late spring, there are usually baby goats, or kids, frolicking around the barnyard. In 1960, the Sandburg's most famous goat, Jennifer II, was internationally recognized for producing 2.5 gallons of milk per day. That's some goat!

Nearby Attractions

The Flat Rock Playhouse, the state theater of North Carolina, is directly opposite the Carl Sandburg Home National Historic Site on Little River Road. Visit flatrockplayhouse.org or call 828-693-0731 for information and tickets. Directly to the southwest of the Little River Road/NC 225 intersection, there is a quaint conglomeration of shops in the heart of historic Flat Rock. After the hike, consider eating lunch in one of the local eateries, then shopping for a unique gift at the eclectic stores that line NC 225.

Directions

Travel I-26 south from Asheville to Exit 53. Turn right off the exit onto Upward Road. Travel 1.2 miles and come to a traffic light at US 176. Continue straight across US 176, at which point the road becomes North Highland Lake Road. Travel North Highland Lake Road 1.1 miles until it dead-ends at NC 225. Turn left onto NC 225 and travel 0.8 mile to a traffic light at the intersection with Little River Road. Turn right onto Little River Road, and in 300 yards turn left into the Carl Sandburg Home National Historic Site.

A GOAT RESTS OUTSIDE THE BARN AT CONNEMARA FARMS.

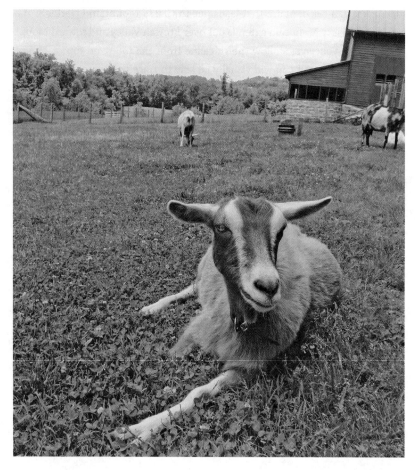

22

DuPont State Forest Four Falls

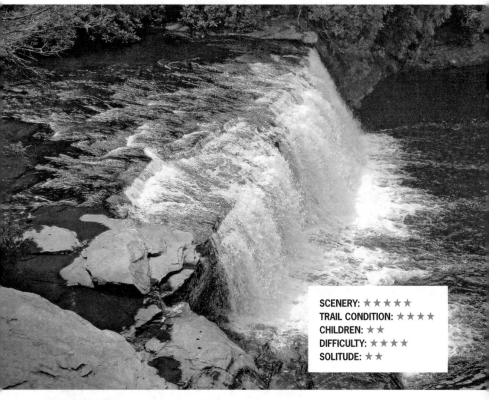

SCENERY: ★ ★ ★ ★ ★
TRAIL CONDITION: ★ ★ ★ ★
CHILDREN: ★ ★
DIFFICULTY: ★ ★ ★ ★
SOLITUDE: ★ ★

HOOKER FALLS

TRAILHEAD GPS COORDINATES: 35.203083, -82.618950

DISTANCE & CONFIGURATION: 9-mile balloon

HIKING TIME: 4.5 hours

HIGHLIGHTS: Four dramatic mountain waterfalls

ELEVATION: 2,216' at trailhead, 2,588' at covered bridge

ACCESS: Free; open daily, 5 a.m.–10 p.m.

MAPS: National Geographic #504 *DuPont State Recreational Forest*; USGS *Brevard, Standingstone Mountain*

FACILITIES: Restrooms at the Hooker Falls Trailhead

WHEELCHAIR ACCESS: None

COMMENTS: This hike can be shortened to 5.4 miles by skipping the out-and-back portion to Bridal Veil Falls.

CONTACTS: 828-877-6527, dupontstaterecreationalforest.com

DuPont State Forest Four Falls

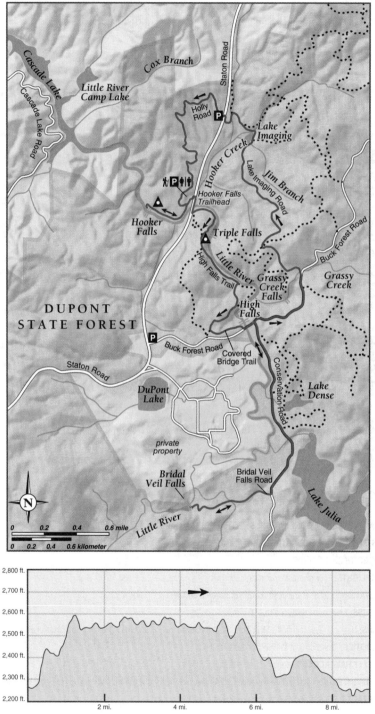

Overview

If you like waterfalls, then you will love this hike. Within the first 1.5 miles, you will see Triple Falls and High Falls, two of the most stunning cataracts in the Southeast. Past High Falls, you will travel into the heart of DuPont State Forest to visit Bridal Veil Falls. After Bridal Veil Falls, you will then backtrack before veering east to visit Lake Imaging. After leaving the lake, you will hike to within sight of the trailhead, where you began, before completing a quick out-and-back to the final cascade, Hooker Falls.

Route Details

In northern DuPont State Forest, you begin this 9-mile balloon hike at the Hooker Falls Trailhead, in the Hooker Falls parking area. Although you may see several people in the parking area hiking west to the namesake nearby water-fall, resist the urge to follow them. Hooker Falls will serve as your finale for this adventure. Instead, to begin your journey, carefully cross Staton Road and walk over the bridge that spans the Little River.

Once on the other side of the river, step over the guardrail at the Triple Falls Trailhead. There you will briefly dip to the banks of the river and then immediately begin a steep ascent. Every uphill footstep is worth it, when in 0.5 mile you arrive at the Triple Falls overlook. The view is spectacular. A pavilion to the right allows you to sit and enjoy the view, while a trail to the left leads down to the base of the falls. When you are finally ready to move on, hike another few dozen yards uphill and turn left (southwest) on High Falls Trail.

High Falls Trail parallels Little River. At 1 mile, a clearing on the left side of the trail provides the best view of the cascade, which is just as breathtaking as Triple Falls. From this viewpoint you will notice that, above the falls, a quaint covered bridge crowns the rushing currents of water. Here is the story behind that:

Back in 1999, High Falls, Triple Falls, and Bridal Veil Falls were part of a spectacular high-profile, two-year land controversy. A local developer bought a large tract, which included the three waterfalls, and started to develop the property into a private community. The developer got as far as building the beautiful, covered bridge that spans High Falls and putting in many of the gravel roads that now serve as DuPont State Forest trails; but before the lots on the property were divided and sold, the state intervened and used the right of eminent domain to buy the land from the developer.

To the delight of conservationists, this act protected the land and the waterfalls. It also made the natural resource available to the general public, as opposed to the few who would have lived in the community. However, many citizens will still argue that the government overstepped its bounds by forcibly taking the property. Still, it's yours to enjoy now.

Past the High Falls lookout, hike another 0.2 mile and then veer left (east) onto the Covered Bridge Trail. This path leads to Buck Forest Road and the west entrance of the covered bridge. Turn left onto Buck Forest Road and walk through the covered bridge. Then turn right onto Conservation Road. Follow Conservation Road 1.5 miles through a diverse forest of maple, long-needle pine, Fraser magnolia, and beech trees.

Beside the road, the forest opens up to reveal pastures and a barn. When you have reached that setting, turn right onto Bridal Veil Falls Road. Follow the road 0.5 mile to the third waterfall of the hike. If you travel along the banks to the upper portion of Bridal Veil Falls, it may look familiar to you. That is because this waterfall was used for one of the scenes in the popular 1992 movie *The Last of the Mohicans*. Most of this epic film was shot in Western North Carolina, near Chimney Rock and Lake Lure, but the scene in which the main characters walk behind a cascading wall of water took place at Bridal Veil Falls.

The rocky riverbank at the base of the falls provides a nice place to sit underneath the shade of an evergreen tree. Once rested up, begin backtracking to the covered bridge via Bridal Veil Falls Road and Conservation Road.

At the covered bridge, turn right, away from High Falls, onto Buck Forest Road. Travel down this gravel pathway 0.6 mile and then turn left onto Lake Imaging Road. (In a few hundred yards, you will notice a trail on your left leading to Grassy Creek Falls. Although the Grassy Creek waterfall does not have the same volume as the previous three cascades, it is a pleasant side destination.)

After walking nearly 8 miles and seeing so much rushing water, it will be a welcome relief to see the still surface of Lake Imaging. Take a minute to rest near the shore of this lake, which was named for the film-processing plant located farther upstream, and then continue through the parking lot. Exit at Lake Imaging Trailhead and cross Staton Road. Turn right and walk on the shoulder of the road about 70 yards until you reach the Holly Road Trailhead.

Turn right onto Holly Road and follow it through a forest of holly trees, poplars, and rhododendrons. During the warmer months, in some sections you might also notice a thick carpet of lycopodium lining the trail.

Follow Holly Road until just before the Hooker Falls parking area, and then turn right onto Hooker Falls Road. A quick 0.8-mile out-and-back jaunt on this path will take you to the last of the four waterfalls on this hike. Hooker Falls is a short and wide waterfall and offers a nice finale to such a spectacular hike, as well as a superlative swimming hole.

Directions

From I-26 take Exit 40 and turn right onto NC 280 toward Brevard. Travel NC 280 south 16 miles to the intersection with US 64. Turn right onto US 64 West and drive 3.7 miles to Crab Creek Road. At Crab Creek Road, turn left and travel 4.3 miles to the intersection with DuPont Road. Take a right onto DuPont Road. Shortly after taking DuPont Road, watch for a name change to Staton Road. The Hooker Falls Trailhead and parking area are 3.1 miles ahead on the right.

23 Lake Julia

SCENERY: ★ ★ ★ ★
TRAIL CONDITION: ★ ★ ★ ★
CHILDREN: ★ ★
DIFFICULTY: ★ ★ ★ ★ ★
SOLITUDE: ★ ★ ★ ★

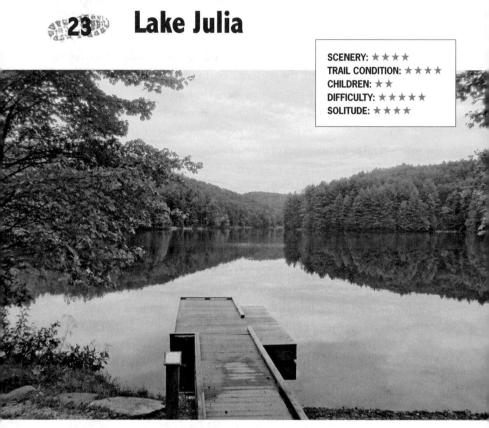

A WOODEN DOCK STRETCHES INTO THE WATER AT LAKE JULIA.

TRAILHEAD GPS COORDINATES: 35.172799, -82.638895

DISTANCE & CONFIGURATION: 10-mile balloon

HIKING TIME: 5 hours

HIGHLIGHTS: Fording Little River and great views of Lake Julia

ELEVATION: 2,708' at trailhead, 3,051' on top of Mine Mountain

ACCESS: Free; open daily, 5 a.m.–10 p.m.

MAPS: National Geographic #504 *DuPont State Recreational Forest*; USGS *Brevard, Standingstone Mountain*

FACILITIES: None

WHEELCHAIR ACCESS: None

COMMENTS: This hike includes a river crossing, which must be forded at the beginning and end of the hike. The route should not be attempted by those uncomfortable in water or unable to swim. In normal conditions the water depth will not exceed 1.5 feet, but water levels and current can vary dramatically based on rainfall. River shoes with good traction are recommended, as the rocks are very slick.

CONTACTS: 828-877-6527, ncforestservice.gov

Overview

This route travels through the remote southern portion of DuPont State Forest, and the ford across the Little River limits foot traffic in this area. When the leaves are off the trees, the ensuing climb of Laurel Ridge and Mine Mountain will reveal views of Pisgah National Forest to the north. The hike then wanders along the banks of Reasonover Creek to reach the shore of beautiful Lake Julia before returning to the trailhead through a hardwood forest.

Route Details

Instead of starting at the popular Hooker Falls or Buck Forest Trailheads, this hike begins at the more remote Corn Mill Shoals parking lot. By starting in the southern portion of the forest, you will avoid the crowds that come to DuPont State Forest to view the waterfalls.

The hike begins by crossing Cascade Lake Road onto Corn Mill Shoals Road. Corn Mill Shoals Road is a narrow gravel road that is closed to traffic. You will travel on this wide, rocky path for about a mile. Along the way you will pass several spur trails that veer off of this main DuPont artery, but you will want to stay on the main path until you reach the Little River. When you arrive at the Little River, you may wonder whether or not you missed a turn, but—for the adventurous hiker—this is not a dead end. It is a river ford!

When the water is at medium or low levels, the crossing appears to be non-technical and shallow. But because the rocks are very slick and the water is moving quickly, you should not attempt this ford if you are not an experienced and sure-footed hiker. Hiking poles help enormously in situations such as this. The recommended method for crossing this river is to put on appropriate water shoes with good traction, and then cross a little upstream of the trail. A few steps to the south will provide slower-flowing water and more bottom debris, which provides a better grip. If you are wearing a day pack, be sure to unbuckle your straps before crossing the water. Should you slip, you will not want to be weighed down by a cumbersome pack. Depending on recent rains, you can anticipate the water to reach no higher than your kneecaps, and it should take you about 10 minutes to change footwear, adjust your pack, and successfully ford the river.

When you reach the opposite shore, you will discover that you are once again on Corn Mill Shoals Road. Follow this trail another 100 yards, and then

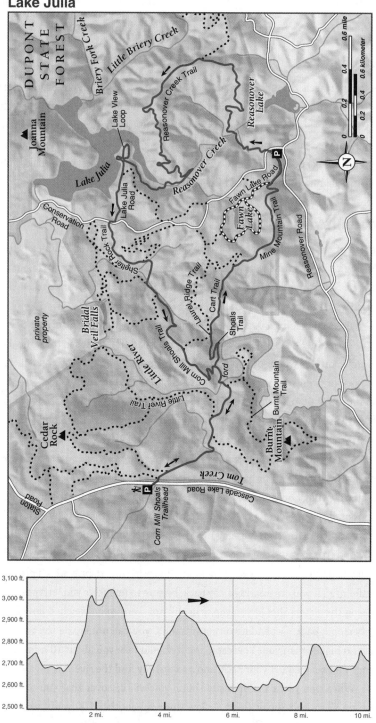

turn right onto Shoals Trail. This narrow path presents a strenuous 0.5-mile climb on a path bordered with fern varieties such as lady finger and Christmas ferns.

When you reach the ridge, veer right onto Laurel Ridge Trail. The next 1.5 miles will parallel the southern boundary of the forest on several adjoining trails. DuPont can often feel very confusing because of the short intersecting trails, but, thankfully, most of the intersections are very well marked. Always bring a map when hiking at DuPont and download one on your phone for good measure.

After 0.1 mile on Laurel Ridge Trail, veer right (east) onto Cart Trail; in another 0.4 mile, veer right again onto Mine Mountain Trail. From the spine of Mine Mountain, you can look to the north and view the neighboring blue ridges of Pisgah National Forest.

When Mine Mountain Trail terminates, turn right (east) onto Fawn Lake Road. Stay straight on the gravel road. In another 0.1 mile the road changes names and becomes known as Reasonover Creek Trail. Follow Reasonover Creek Trail through a mixed forest of long-needle pines, oaks, Fraser magnolias, and sassafras. This is one of the least-traveled paths in the forest and provides several fallen trees and rocks on which to sit and enjoy the silence and surrounding solitude.

At 3.6 miles the path crosses Reasonover Creek on several strategically placed rocks. (After experiencing wet feet for yourself at the Little River ford, you will especially appreciate the work of the trail crew who positioned these large rocks in the creek.) After 3.3 miles Reasonover Creek Trail terminates at Lake Julia.

A scenic mountain lake, Julia originally was created for water sports at Camp Summit, a coed children's summer destination for more than two decades. On the hike back to the trailhead you could take a short detour and visit the landing strip that was put in for the camp owner's small aircraft.

For the best views of the lake, travel on the short 0.2-mile Lake View Loop. When you are ready to leave the waterfront, follow Lake Julia Road to Conservation Road. At Conservation Road, turn right and then take an immediate left onto Shelter Rock Trail. Follow Shelter Rock Trail to Corn Mill Shoals Trail, and then travel Corn Mill Shoals Road back to the Little River. You will need to ford the water one more time to make it back to the parking lot. Remember that you are more tired now than at the beginning of your hike, so be extra cautious on this crossing.

When you are safely on the other shoreline, continue on Corn Mill Shoals Road another mile to the Corn Mill Shoals parking lot.

Directions

From I-26 take Exit 40 and turn right onto NC 280 toward Brevard. Travel NC 280 south 16 miles to the intersection with US 64. Turn right onto US 64 West and drive 3.7 miles to Crab Creek Road. At Crab Creek Road, turn left and travel 4.3 miles to the intersection with DuPont Road. Take a right onto DuPont Road. Shortly after taking DuPont Road, watch for a name change to Staton Road. After 5.3 miles the road will terminate at an intersection with Cascade Lake Road. Turn left on Cascade Lake Road. Drive 0.8 mile to the Corn Mill Shoals parking area on the right.

STEPPING-STONES AID YOUR CROSSING OF REASONOVER CREEK.

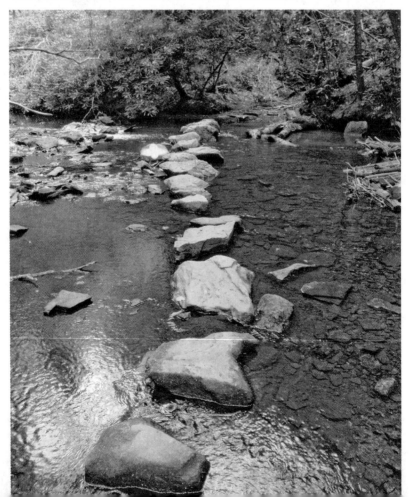

John Rock

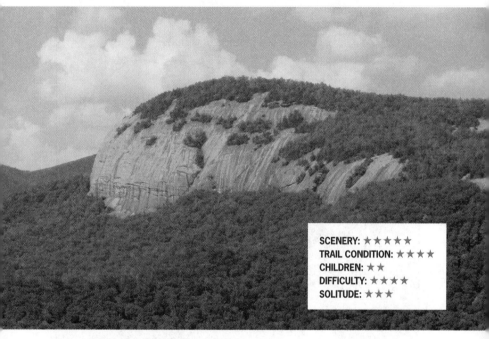

SCENERY: ★ ★ ★ ★ ★
TRAIL CONDITION: ★ ★ ★ ★
CHILDREN: ★ ★
DIFFICULTY: ★ ★ ★ ★
SOLITUDE: ★ ★ ★

A VIEW OF LOOKING GLASS ROCK FROM JOHN ROCK

TRAILHEAD GPS COORDINATES: 35.284166, -82.790660

DISTANCE & CONFIGURATION: 6-mile loop

HIKING TIME: 3.5 hours

HIGHLIGHTS: Great views of Looking Glass Rock and Pisgah National Forest

ELEVATION: 2,318' at trailhead, 3,200' on top of John Rock

ACCESS: Free and always open

MAPS: National Geographic #780 *Pisgah Ranger District;* USGS *Shining Rock*

FACILITIES: Restrooms, a gift shop, and trailside museum at the wildlife education center

WHEELCHAIR ACCESS: Yes, at the wildlife education center

CONTACTS: Pisgah National Forest, Pisgah Ranger District, 828-877-3265, fs.usda.gov/nfsnc

Overview

From the Pisgah fish hatchery, the route follows Cat Gap Loop Trail across Cedar Rock Creek and then travels beside the creek to reach Cedar Rock Falls. Leaving the creek, the path continues uphill and passes through multiple hemlock

John Rock

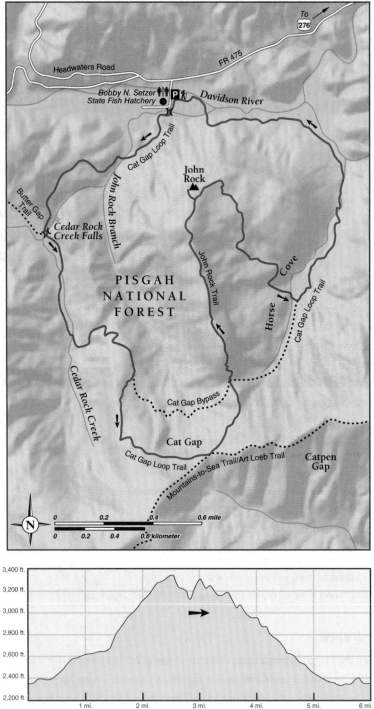

groves to reach John Rock Trail. After climbing over the top of John Rock, you will see a marked side trail that leads to an exposed rock and panoramic overlook. Enjoy viewing the west slopes of Looking Glass Mountain, and then return to the John Rock Trail and follow it downhill to rejoin Cat Gap Loop Trail and conclude the hike.

Route Details

When driving into the parking lot for the Bobby N. Setzer State Fish Hatchery and the John Rock Trailhead, you will notice a large bronze statue to your right. This monument is dedicated to the men in the Civilian Conservation Corps (CCC) who were stationed at Camp John Rock. Between 1933 and 1941, the level area of land that is now home to the parking lot, former wildlife education center, and fish hatchery was a work camp for young men employed to complete federal projects in Pisgah National Forest, such as the Blue Ridge Parkway.

With its proximity to the clear waters of the Davidson River and terrific view of John Rock, the appeal of the level terrain is easy to appreciate. In fact, before the land was utilized by the CCC, it was used as a logging camp, and later it became home to a Boy Scout camp. Today, it is fortunate that the area is open to the general public.

When you are ready to locate the trail, follow the paved road in the southwest corner of the parking area. If you are facing the front of the former wildlife education center it will be the road directly to your left. As you walk down the road, you will notice a fence to your left and a Forest Service gate that bars vehicles. Step around the gate and then look for a bridge across Cedar Rock Creek to your right. Cross over the bridge and turn right (southwest) onto the red-blazed Cat Gap Loop Trail.

Once you are on Cat Gap Loop Trail, you will hike a moderate ascent through a dense forest of towering tulip poplars and oaks mixed with thick rhododendron and mountain laurel. At 0.8 mile you will notice a large, frequently used campsite by the banks of Cedar Rock Creek. There is a hidden waterfall near this campsite, known as Cedar Rock Creek Falls. To view the cascade, hike down to the flat tent spots, and then follow the banks of the river 20 yards upstream. Be cautious to avoid slipping on any wet roots or rocks.

Past the waterfall, the trail continues to gain elevation to reach nearby Butter Gap. There, you will need to walk carefully over a log bridge that spans the creek and then turn right (southeast). Stay on Cat Gap Loop Trail and follow the red blazes through a green mountain laurel tunnel. In this section of Pisgah National Forest, the pink-white blooms of the mountain laurel trees usually open in late May. And they are closely followed by the pink and purple rhododendron flowers.

The path remains close to Cedar Rock Creek, and at 1.3 miles you will have to once again cross it, this time by rock-hopping on large stones. When the trail comes to the Cat Gap Bypass intersection, at 1.8 miles, stay straight and hike uphill to remain on Cat Gap Loop Trail.

Your steady uphill climb concludes at Cat Gap, where the Cat Gap Loop Trail briefly touches but does not cross the white-blazed Art Loeb Trail before veering left and descending the ridge. This short downhill serves as a brief respite, but there is still a little bit of climbing to the lookout at John Rock. After hiking 2.4 miles, you will arrive at a four-way intersection: continue straight

THE FISH HATCHERY IS TO THE LEFT, WHILE LOOKING GLASS ROCK IS PARTLY SHROUDED IN CLOUD COVER.

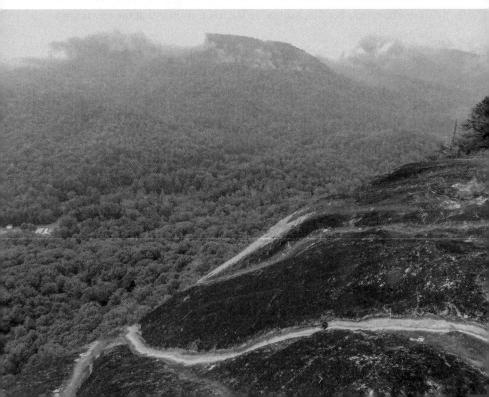

and hike uphill on the John Rock Trail. You will soon reach the hike's highest point of elevation at 3,200 feet. From there, travel one more undulating climb and then, at 3.5 miles, follow the John Rock spur trail to your left.

The view from John Rock offers a dramatic profile of Looking Glass Rock to the east and a panoramic view of the Pisgah Ridge to the north. Directly below you can see the trout pools at the fish hatchery, and possibly even your car in the parking lot. Always remember to be very careful on the exposed granite, as it is a steep 200-foot drop to the rocks below. Take extra caution if there has been recent rain or ice.

Beyond John Rock, the trail descends to rejoin Cat Gap Loop Trail at 4.3 miles. Turn left on Cat Gap Loop Trail and follow the relatively level trail through a forest that is defined by tall, straight poplar trees. After 4.8 miles the trail intersects a gravel road and then crosses over two streambeds. As you near the conclusion of your hike, you will parallel the Davidson River, and you may be able to watch a fly fisherman testing his luck. Many of the trout that live in the water were raised at the nearby fish hatchery. You may want to consider visiting the fish hatchery after exiting the forest at the northeast end of the parking lot.

Nearby Attractions

After your hike, consider visiting the Bobby N. Setzer State Fish Hatchery. Visit ncwildlife.org or call 828-877-4423 to learn more.

Directions

From Asheville, take I-26 to Exit 40, the Asheville Airport and Brevard Road/NC 280 exit. Turn right off the exit and follow NC 280 for 17 miles to the outskirts of Brevard. At the US 64/US 276 intersection, turn right and enter Pisgah National Forest. Continue 5.5 miles on US 276 and then turn left onto Forest Road 475. The Bobby N. Setzer State Fish Hatchery and John Rock Trailhead will be 1.5 miles on your left.

25 **Looking Glass Rock**

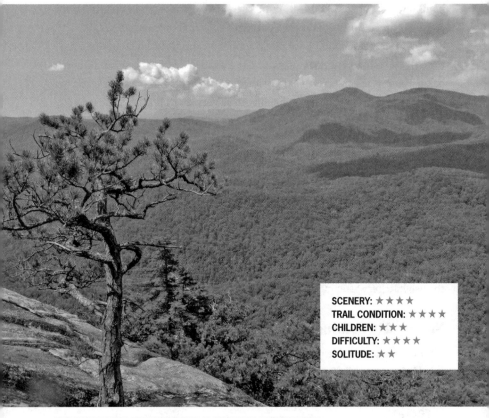

SCENERY: ★ ★ ★ ★
TRAIL CONDITION: ★ ★ ★ ★
CHILDREN: ★ ★ ★
DIFFICULTY: ★ ★ ★ ★
SOLITUDE: ★ ★

THE PANORAMAS FROM LOOKING GLASS ROCK ARE AMAZING!

TRAILHEAD GPS COORDINATES: 35.290883, -82.776517

DISTANCE & CONFIGURATION: 6-mile out-and-back

HIKING TIME: 3.5 hours

HIGHLIGHTS: Beautiful views of Pisgah Ridge from the top of Looking Glass Rock

ELEVATION: 2,303' at the trailhead, 3,960' just above Looking Glass Rock

ACCESS: Free and always open

MAPS: National Geographic #780 *Pisgah Ranger District;* USGS *Shining Rock*

FACILITIES: None

COMMENTS: Be aware that there is a steep drop near the edge of Looking Glass Rock. Stay near the path and trees to enjoy the view.

CONTACTS: Pisgah National Forest, Pisgah Ranger District, 828-877-3265, fs.usda.gov/nfsnc

Overview

Looking Glass Rock is one of the most recognized natural features in Western North Carolina. For many motorists who travel the Blue Ridge Parkway, viewing the giant monolith is one of the highlights of their trip. However, to actually hike to the top of the granite rock face, you will have to take a narrow trail up multiple switchbacks to reach the ridge of Looking Glass Rock. There, you will enjoy some relatively level hiking before the trail offers a brief descent that places you directly on top of Looking Glass Rock. From this overlook, you will enjoy fantastic north-facing views.

Route Details

Back in a time unknown, continental plates beneath the Earth's surface collided, causing tension and heat to melt sedimentary rock into magma. That magma solidified into Whiteside granite, and today Looking Glass Rock provides stunning views of the eroded rock. Geologically classified as a pluton monolith, Looking Glass Rock gained its name from the bright reflection of sunlight off of its exposed granite.

Rising over 1,700 feet from the valley floor, Looking Glass Rock is a popular destination for both hikers and mountain climbers. To get to the top of the steep granite slope, start at the Looking Glass parking area and trailhead off Forest Road 475, hike west from the only trailhead in the parking area, then continue to veer left onto a well-defined singletrack trail, and begin your ascent.

Early on, the climb is moderate and contours the hillside above a small stream coursing down Looking Glass Rock. However, after hiking 0.4 mile you will begin a long stretch of switchbacks that slowly weave their way up the mountain. The twisting, turning trail winds through a hardwood forest of tulip poplar, Fraser magnolia, hickory, sourwood, and beech trees.

After hiking a little over a mile uphill, you will arrive at a small rock outcrop. By taking a few steps off the path to explore this overlook, you will be able to view the mountains and ridges to the east and north. During the winter months it is possible to identify Bearpen Mountain and Coontree Mountain from this spot. There is also a twisted root formation sprawling out across the granite overlook that is almost as rewarding to study as the view.

Looking Glass Rock

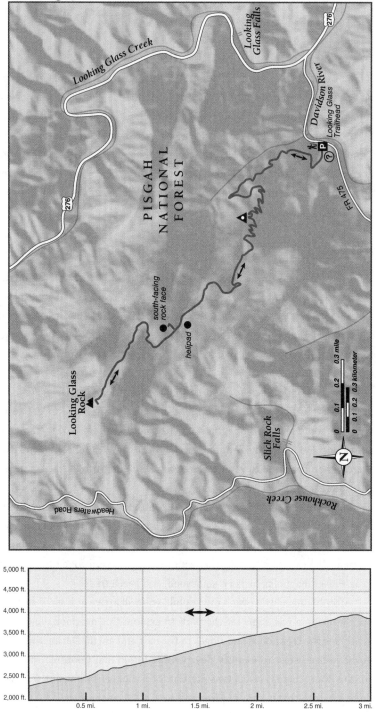

At 1.4 miles you will enter a dense rhododendron patch. When you exit the long green tunnel, you will be greeted with a more level grade and an end to the switchbacks. Although you are no longer weaving your way up the side of the mountain, you still gradually gain elevation on your way to Looking Glass Ridge. At 2 miles you will notice an exposed area of level granite bordering the trail. This serves as a helipad to rescue injured hikers or climbers in the area.

A few hundred yards beyond the helipad, you will notice a slanted rock wall on your right. If you take the time to climb to the top of this steep exposed granite, you will be rewarded with terrific southern views that are not available from Looking Glass Rock. The vista even provides glimpses of two neighboring pluton monoliths: John Rock and Cedar Rock Mountain.

After leaving this viewpoint, continue along the ridge amid the copious galax that lines the trail. At 2.7 miles you will reach a campsite on top of Looking Glass Mountain, but in order to access the incredible views from the top of the exposed rock face, you will need to travel another 0.1 mile slightly downhill to where the forest opens up on top of the giant monolith.

On a clear day, the view from on top of Looking Glass Rock reveals Pisgah Ridge and the Blue Ridge Parkway to the north. This is also a popular spot for ravens to soar directly above the rock, and seasonally you might also notice a threatened peregrine falcon coming to roost in the rocky ledges. An even stranger sight might be watching a person or two appear over the edge of the vertical north slope of the mountain.

It may seem implausible for someone to access the summit from the north side of the mountain, but this is a favorite destination for many skilled mountain climbers. The sheer rock face of Looking Glass provides several different climbing routes to the summit. You may be tempted to walk closer to the edge and watch these individuals climb the mountain or look for a peregrine falcon nest below, but remember that you are not attached to a rope or a harness, so do not travel too far from the edge of the forest.

When you are ready to say goodbye to the beautiful views from the top of Looking Glass Rock, retrace your steps slightly uphill for a few hundred yards to the mountaintop campsite, and then enjoy an entirely downhill trip back to the parking area.

Nearby Attractions

If you head southeast from the trailhead, the Bobby N. Setzer State Fish Hatchery is 1 mile farther down FR 475 on the left. The hatchery is open to the public during normal working hours, 8 a.m.–4 p.m., on weekdays.

Directions

From Asheville, take I-26 to Exit 40, the Asheville Airport and Brevard Road/NC 280 exit. Turn right off the exit and follow NC 280 for 17 miles to the outskirts of Brevard. At the US 64/US 276 intersection, turn right and enter Pisgah National Forest. Continue on US 276 for 5.5 miles and then turn left onto FR 475. Drive 0.4 mile and then turn into the Looking Glass parking lot on the right.

YOU CAN TAKE IN A GREAT VIEW OF PISGAH RIDGE FROM LOOKING GLASS ROCK.

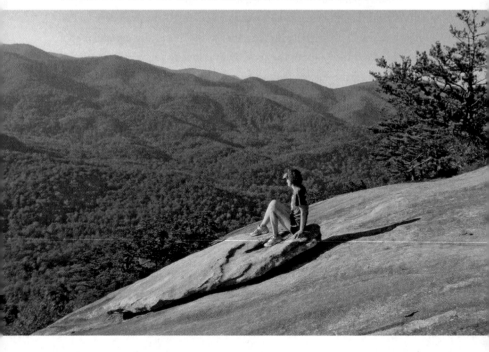

Moore Cove Falls

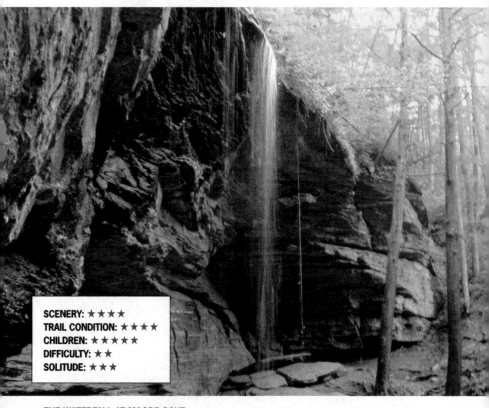

SCENERY: ★ ★ ★ ★
TRAIL CONDITION: ★ ★ ★ ★
CHILDREN: ★ ★ ★ ★ ★
DIFFICULTY: ★ ★
SOLITUDE: ★ ★ ★

THE WATERFALL AT MOORE COVE

TRAILHEAD GPS COORDINATES: 35.305489, -82.774636

DISTANCE & CONFIGURATION: 1.4-mile out-and-back

HIKING TIME: 1 hour

HIGHLIGHTS: A 50-foot vertical waterfall

ELEVATION: 2,555' at trailhead, 2,667' near Moore Cove Falls

ACCESS: Free and always open

MAPS: National Geographic #780 *Pisgah Ranger District;* USGS *Shining Rock*

FACILITIES: None

WHEELCHAIR ACCESS: None

COMMENTS: This waterfall is perfect for standing underneath if you can bear the cold water, but beware of slick rocks and do not try to climb to the top of the falls.

CONTACTS: Pisgah National Forest, Pisgah Ranger District, 828-877-3265, fs.usda.gov/nfsnc

Moore Cove Falls

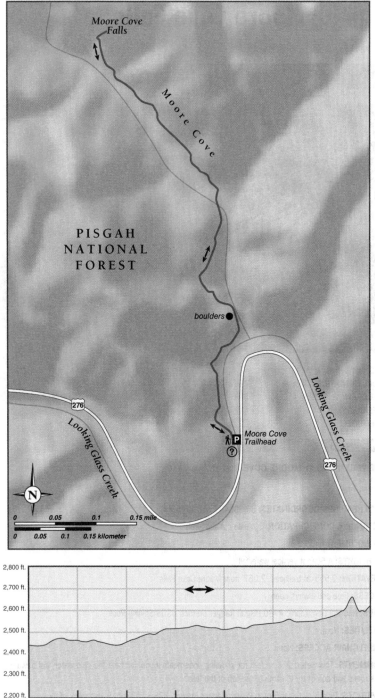

Overview

The short, scenic Moore Cove hike leads you across Looking Glass Creek and through a forest dominated by tulip poplar, beech, and other hardwoods. The route weaves between two large boulders on either side of the trail and then traverses several footbridges before arriving at the 50-foot Moore Cove Falls. On a hot summer day, many hikers like to cool off in the waterfall's refreshing shower and cold stream before backtracking to the trailhead.

Route Details

This under-the-radar hike is located between two of the most well-known waterfalls in Western North Carolina, Looking Glass Falls and Sliding Rock. You will pass Looking Glass Falls on your drive to Moore Cove Falls. You can view the dramatic cascade from the road or travel down a few dozen steps to stand near the base of the falls. This outing can be turned into a waterfall extravaganza by stopping to enjoy the views at Looking Glass, hiking in to scenic and kid-friendly Moore Cove Falls, and then ending the day by taking a few trips down nature's waterslide at Sliding Rock.

To begin the hike, locate the wooden kiosk that serves as the trailhead at the Moore Cove parking area. From the kiosk, travel across Looking Glass Creek on the wooden bridge. Looking Glass Creek is the mother stream for stunning Looking Glass Falls a few miles farther down. After falling over the 60-foot vertical drop at Looking Glass Falls, the creek then winds its way down the mountain to meet the Davidson River, a tributary of the French Broad River, which is, in turn, a tributary of the Tennessee River.

After passing over Looking Glass Creek, watch for the trail blazes and follow them up a slight incline into a forest lined with tulip poplar and beech trees. The trail levels out for a brief period, and then, at 0.2 mile, you will walk down a brief descent that ends between two large boulders. These large boulders seem misplaced, without any other rock formations or rock fields nearby, but they certainly offer an intriguing spot to rest in the shade.

If you do stop at the boulders, you may also want to observe more closely the mountain laurel bushes that seemingly grow atop the boulders, and then trace their sprawling root system to see where they are finding their nutrients. You may discover that most of the roots are actually planted in soft earth, but over time the body of the tree has migrated out over the rock to receive more sunlight.

After passing through the boulders, you will come to a small stream. A faint rabbit trail to the right leads beside the stream, but you will want to continue straight on the main path and cross over the stream. You will crisscross this stream several times on your way to Moore Cove Falls. Be extra careful if conditions are slick, as the trail can become muddy and the log bridges can become treacherous in wet weather.

Now that the path closely parallels the small stream, you will notice that the undergrowth beside the trail becomes especially dense and verdant. The moisture-rich habitat is home to doghobble and several different varieties of ferns. You might also spot a patch of heart-shaped leaves growing on individual stems, very close to the ground. This is wild ginger. It is not related to the pickled pink root that is served beside your sushi, but it does have a similar smell and taste. And, although technically edible, wild ginger is not used to flavor food because of the plant's diuretic properties.

MOUNTAIN LAURELS GROW ATOP THE BOULDERS ON THE TRAIL.

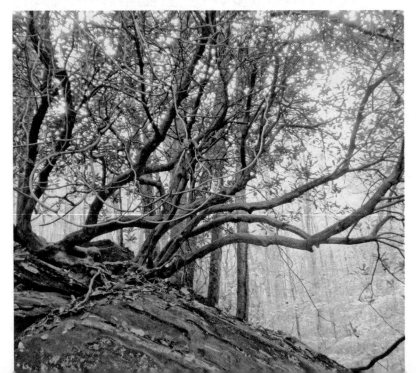

At 0.7 mile you will hike up a slight incline away from the creekbed to the crest of a hill, where you are rewarded with views of Moore Cove Falls. The thin stream of water falling off the red-tinted cliffs makes a 50-foot journey to reach the slick rocks below. Compared with its neighbor, Looking Glass Falls, Moore Cove Falls looks more like a trickle than a waterfall. But unlike Looking Glass, the delicate stream of Moore Cove Falls allows you to get closer to the action. Worn footpaths surround the cascade. You can walk behind the waterfall, in front of the waterfall, or beside the waterfall, and on a hot day, many people choose to walk directly under the waterfall.

As you explore the falls, remember that many of the rocks are worn and slick, so take extra caution with your foot placement. And, as recommended by the Forest Service, do not try to hike to the top of the falls.

After leaving Moore Cove Falls and backtracking to the parking lot, you may want to consider visiting Sliding Rock before heading home—especially if you are already wet.

Nearby Attractions

Drive 1 mile north on US 276 to find the entrance of Sliding Rock on your left. For a small parking fee, you can enjoy as many trips as you care to take down nature's waterslide. The fast-moving water, smooth rock, and gentle grade carry you swiftly downstream to a pool at the bottom of the rock. Water shoes and shorts or pants are recommended. Sliding Rock is open and staffed, during daylight hours, with lifeguards on duty early May through mid-September.

Directions

From Asheville, take I-26 to Exit 40, the Asheville Airport and Brevard Road/NC 280 exit. Turn right off the exit and follow NC 280 for 17 miles to the outskirts of Brevard. At the US 64/US 276 intersection, turn right onto US 276 and enter Pisgah National Forest. Continue 6.6 miles on US 276. The parking area for Moore Cove is located directly off the right shoulder of the road, just before the highway crosses a bridge over Looking Glass Creek. There are no visible signs that designate the Moore Cove Trailhead from the road, but you will be able to spot a wooden information kiosk near the footbridge.

Turkey Pen Loop

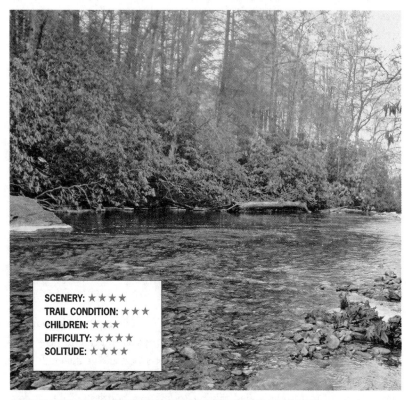

TURKEY PEN LOOP INCLUDES A FORD OF THE SOUTH FORK MILLS RIVER.

SCENERY: ★ ★ ★ ★
TRAIL CONDITION: ★ ★ ★
CHILDREN: ★ ★ ★
DIFFICULTY: ★ ★ ★ ★
SOLITUDE: ★ ★ ★ ★

TRAILHEAD GPS COORDINATES: 35.342905, -82.659421

DISTANCE & CONFIGURATION: 4.6-mile loop

HIKING TIME: 2.5 hours

HIGHLIGHTS: South Mills River

ELEVATION: 2,378' at the river, 2,780' at Mullinax Trail intersection

ACCESS: Free and always open

MAPS: National Geographic #780 *Pisgah Ranger District;* USGS *Pisgah National Forest*

FACILITIES: None

WHEELCHAIR ACCESS: None

COMMENTS: This hike includes a river ford and should not be attempted by those uncomfortable in water or unable to swim. In normal conditions the water depth will not exceed 2 feet, but water levels and current can vary.

CONTACTS: Pisgah National Forest, Pisgah Ranger District, 828-877-3265, fs.usda.gov/nfsnc

Overview

This hike will take you through the heart of Turkey Pen in Pisgah National Forest. The route begins by contouring the banks of the South Fork Mills River. After 1.2 miles you will be faced with a chilly, adventurous, adult knee–level river ford. Continuing on with wet feet, you will travel on rolling terrain through a peaceful hardwood forest. Near the end of the hike, the trail will descend to the South Fork Mills River, and you will need to cross the rushing water once again. This time, however, a suspension bridge spares you another river ford; by the time you return to the trailhead, you will have a smile on your face, lots of pictures on your phone, and maybe even dry feet!

Route Details

Turkey Pen is a hidden hiking gem in Pisgah National Forest. Tucked between North Mills River Recreation Area and Brevard, the area is one of the most popular horseback riding destinations in Pisgah. The rough road leading to the trailhead and the river fords, even the one via the suspension bridge, sometimes discourage hikers and mountain bikers from exploring the terrain. But if you have decent clearance on your car and don't mind getting your feet wet, Turkey Pen Loop offers a great place to seek adventure.

The trails that lead out of the Turkey Pen parking lot offer a wide array of length and difficulty. With trails that connect to Pink Beds, the Pisgah Ranger Station, and the Mountains-to-Sea Trail, this location offers unending day hike and overnight options. That said, before branching out to explore the outer reaches of Turkey Pen, it is important to acquaint yourself with the heart of the trail network. The Turkey Pen Loop does just that. By connecting some of the main pedestrian arteries at Turkey Pen, this hike allows you to become familiar with the terrain and trails at Turkey Pen before choosing to extend your adventure on additional routes.

To begin the Turkey Pen Loop, park in the hiker parking area at the trailhead and locate the wooden information kiosk. (*Note:* Parking in the horse trailer portion of the parking area will result in a fine—unless you happen to have a horse trailer hitched up.)

Once parked, locate the white-blazed South Fork Mills River Trail behind the kiosk to the left of the road. Follow the singletrack trail downhill through a rhododendron tunnel to the bank of the South Fork Mills River.

Turkey Pen Loop

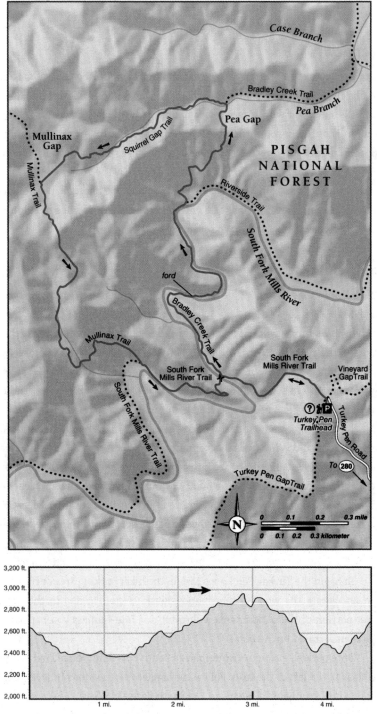

Once you reach the river, at 0.4 mile, you will pass a wooden suspension bridge on your left, and then you will turn right on the orange-blazed Bradley Creek Trail. Continue on Bradley Creek Trail and along the eastern bank of the South Mills River. Several campsites alongside the river provide nice resting spots and good places to play in the water when the temperatures are warm. It is curious that even though you are hiking north, you are still following the river downstream. Mills River is, in fact, part of the French Broad River Basin, and the water will continue to flow north to Hot Springs, North Carolina, and across the Tennessee state line before joining the Tennessee River and eventually heading south to the Gulf of Mexico via the Mississippi River.

After 0.8 mile of walking, you will arrive at what seems to be a dead end when the trail terminates at a sandy riverbank. Upon scanning the forest to the east and to the south, you will clearly see that the trail continues to the north—across the river. It's time to roll up your pants, grab a hiking stick if you aren't equipped with trekking poles, and perhaps remove your socks before braving the cold water and fording. On average, the current is not strong, but the water levels will rise to the knees of an adult. Children may need to be carried across the river. If you feel unsafe fording the river, do not hesitate to turn back to the trailhead at this point.

Once you reach the opposite side of the river, continue the trail on the west bank of the waterway. During the hot summer months, the tall trees and steep slope to the west will provide pleasant shade to walk beneath. The riverbank also offers several protruding rocks, where you can sit and watch the ripples on the surface of the water.

At 1.3 miles arrive at a junction with the Riverside Trail. Turn left at the trail junction and hike uphill and away from the river to remain on Bradley Creek Trail. The trail will lead you through Pea Gap to descend and intersect Squirrel Gap Trail. Turn left on the blue-blazed Squirrel Gap Trail and follow the path on a gradual ascent next to a trickling stream. This portion of the hike is located on the north slope of a ridge that connects Poundingstone Mountain and Buck Mountain. Except for the occasional aircraft, there is very little noise pollution here.

At the west terminus of Squirrel Gap Trail, you will intersect the Mullinax Trail. Turn left on the Mullinax Trail and hike south. At 3 miles the Mullinax Trail makes a sharp left turn (south), and then another sharp turn east at 3.3

miles near a creek crossing. After hiking a cumulative 3.7 miles, the Mullinax Trail ends at a T intersection with the South Mills River Trail. Turn left on the white-blazed South Mills River Trail and follow it across the suspension bridge that spans South Fork Mills River. Beyond the suspension bridge, turn right and retrace your steps back to the Turkey Pen Trailhead.

Directions

Travel I-26 south from Asheville to Exit 40. Turn right off the exit onto NC 280. Continue 11 miles on NC 280. Just past Boyleston Creek Baptist Church, near the Transylvania/Henderson County line, turn right onto Turkey Pen Road. Turkey Pen Road is a narrow, uneven dirt road and is recommended for cars with good clearance. However, passenger cars can make it if driven slowly and carefully. The road conditions improve after you reach the national forest boundary, and after 1.3 miles the road dead-ends at the Turkey Pen parking area and trailhead.

Mills River Loop

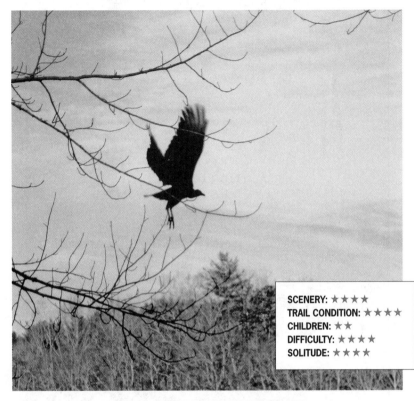

<table>
</table>

SCENERY: ★ ★ ★ ★
TRAIL CONDITION: ★ ★ ★ ★
CHILDREN: ★ ★
DIFFICULTY: ★ ★ ★ ★
SOLITUDE: ★ ★ ★ ★

WILDLIFE IS COPIOUS IN THE NORTH MILLS RIVER RECREATION AREA.

TRAILHEAD GPS COORDINATES: 35.420444, -82.656760

DISTANCE & CONFIGURATION: 8.1-mile loop

HIKING TIME: 4 hours

HIGHLIGHTS: A gentle gradient and scenic forest road

ELEVATION: 2,557' at trailhead, 3,325' on Trace Ridge

ACCESS: Free and always open

MAPS: National Geographic #780 *Pisgah Ranger District*; USGS *Dunsmore Mountain*

FACILITIES: Toilets at North Mills River Recreation Area

WHEELCHAIR ACCESS: None

COMMENTS: The most confusing portion of this hike is getting to the trailhead. Make sure you travel 2.4 miles on the forest road, past a pit toilet and trailhead on your right, to where the road dead-ends at locked U.S. Forest Service gates.

CONTACTS: Pisgah National Forest, Pisgah Ranger District, 828-877-3265, fs.usda.gov/nfsnc

Mills River Loop

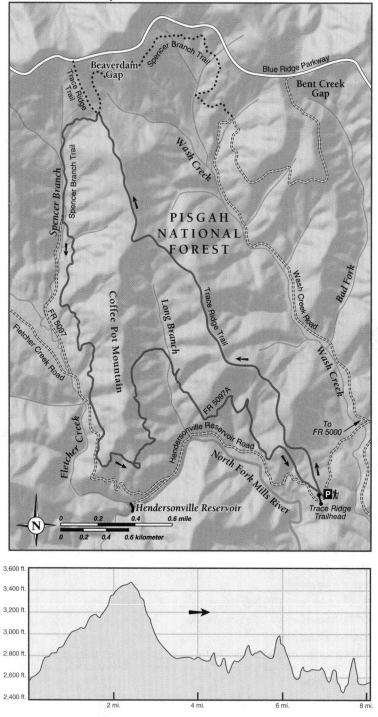

Overview

If you are looking to stretch your legs on a long hike, but at the same time are worried about Western North Carolina's challenging terrain, then this is a great loop to build up your confidence and mileage. You will begin the hike gradually on a singletrack trail along Trace Ridge Trail. Just before reaching the Blue Ridge Parkway, the route descends southeast to meet with Spencer Branch. Past Spencer Branch you will turn left on a normally gated forest road and follow the wide dirt path east. The forest road travels between towering pine and poplar trees and provides an easy stretch of hiking back to the parking lot and trailhead.

Route Details

The Mills River Loop starts at the Trace Ridge Trailhead in the North Mills River Recreation Area. This portion of Pisgah National Forest offers a wealth of connecting trails, and for the ambitious hiker, a longer day hike could lead all the way to Bent Creek—which would add substantial mileage to this route and need to be completed as a shuttle hike as opposed to a loop. This 8.2-mile loop, however, stays near the North Fork Mills River on the south side of Pisgah Ridge.

The route offers a satisfying day hike with gradual grades. The hike is especially inviting in winter, when bare trees reveal views of neighboring mountains and ridgelines.

To begin the hike, locate the gated Forest Road 5097. The gate, to the west of the parking area, marks the beginning and end of the trek. Once you arrive at the gate, do not walk past it, but look to your right and locate the singletrack Trace Ridge Trail. Turn right on the orange-blazed path and follow it uphill into the forest.

After 0.2 mile the singletrack intersects Forest Road 5097A. Follow the combined route 100 yards, and then veer left (west) to continue on Trace Ridge Trail. Follow Trace Ridge Trail back into the forest under a canopy of oak, poplar, and hickory trees. As you continue to make your way uphill, the tall hardwood trees give way to a green tunnel of mountain laurel and rhododendrons. And although you continue to gain elevation, the gentle slope makes the hiking pleasant, and the climb goes almost unnoticed.

At 1.8 miles the trail grade increases, and you will remember that you are, in fact, hiking uphill. For 0.25 mile the trail presents a challenging but manageable ascent and then levels out on the spine of Trace Ridge. At this point you may be able to see or hear the Blue Ridge Parkway to the north. It is hard to imagine that you are so close to the national scenic road because the driving distance between the Blue Ridge Parkway and North Mills River Recreation Area is fairly substantial. However, as the crow flies, you are now less than a mile from the popular motor route.

At 2.7 miles you will notice some loose footing on the treadway, followed by a brief dip in the ridgeline. After traveling the short downhill portion of trail, you will arrive at the Spencer Branch Trail junction. At this point, or at another time, if you wanted to hike to the Blue Ridge Parkway, you could continue straight on the Trace Ridge Trail. However, to continue on this Mills River Loop, you will want to turn left and hike downhill on Spencer Branch Trail.

Your path down Spencer Branch Trail is steep and slightly eroded. At 3.1 miles you will come to Spencer Creek. Rhododendrons, doghobble, and ferns border this small creek. A handful of backcountry campsites and fallen logs near the stream provide a nice resting place to stop and enjoy a snack. The route follows the quaint water source another 0.3 mile to where it crosses under FR 5097. From there the creek will continue down the drainage basin to connect with the North Fork of the Mills River. You, however, will turn east on Forest Road 5097 and contour the slopes of Coffee Pot Mountain.

The winding dirt track provides a scenic route through the tall maple, pine, and Fraser magnolia trees. If you walk quietly, this is an excellent place to spot a deer, wild turkey, or black bear on the slopes below the road. However, because the forest road provides such nice walking and easy access into the depths of the North Mills River Recreation Area, you are also likely to spot a handful of individuals dressed in camouflage. Be sure to wear bright colors if you venture out during hunting season!

At 5.9 miles you will cross over Long Branch, which lines the cove between Coffee Pot Mountain and Trace Ridge. From there you will travel southwest along the mountain slope to the gate at the end of FR 5097, directly to the west of the Trace Ridge Trailhead and your vehicle.

Nearby Attractions

North Mills River Recreation Area offers full-service camping, backcountry campsites, a picnic area, and many opportunities for fly-fishing.

Directions

Travel I-26 south from Asheville to Exit 40. Turn right off the exit onto NC 280 West. Travel 3.9 miles and then turn right on County Road 1345/North Mills River Road and follow it 4.9 miles, then turn right on Forest Road 5000, just before reaching the North Mills River Recreation Area. After 0.3 mile the paved road will give way to packed dirt. At 0.9 mile the road goes around a hairpin turn and continues on to reach a trailhead and road intersection at 1.9 miles. Veer left onto Forest Road 5097 at the intersection and travel across a bridge over Wash Creek. Continue uphill 0.5 mile to reach Trace Ridge Trailhead.

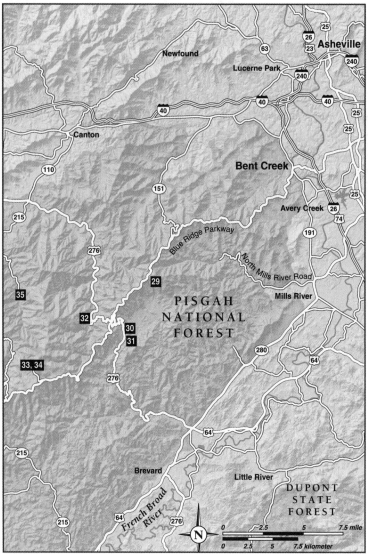

West

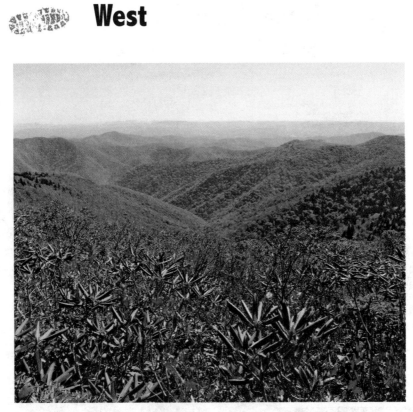

SPECTACULAR VIEWS ARE YOUR REWARD FOR THIS DIFFICULT HIKE *(Hike 32, page 181).*

Mount Pisgah via Buck Spring Lodge

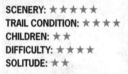

SCENERY: ★ ★ ★ ★ ★
TRAIL CONDITION: ★ ★ ★ ★
CHILDREN: ★ ★
DIFFICULTY: ★ ★ ★ ★
SOLITUDE: ★ ★

MOUNT PISGAH RISES IN ALL ITS GLORY.

TRAILHEAD GPS COORDINATES: 35.403701, -82.753320

DISTANCE & CONFIGURATION: 5.2-mile out-and-back

HIKING TIME: 3 hours

HIGHLIGHTS: The remains of Buck Spring Lodge, George W. Vanderbilt's hunting cabin, and Mount Pisgah's summit and tower

ELEVATION: 4,923' at trailhead, 5,713' at Mount Pisgah's summit

ACCESS: Free and always open, but vehicle access to this hike is unavailable when the Blue Ridge Parkway is closed. Check nps.gov/blri for real-time road closures.

MAPS: National Geographic #780 *Pisgah Ranger District;* USGS *Cruso*

FACILITIES: Restrooms and food located at the Pisgah Inn near the trailhead

WHEELCHAIR ACCESS: None

COMMENTS: Do not let children (or adults) play near the TV tower on the top of Mount Pisgah.

CONTACTS: Blue Ridge Parkway: 828-298-0398, nps.gov/blri; Pisgah National Forest, 828-257-4200, fs.usda.gov/nfsnc

Overview

This hike leads to the top of Mount Pisgah after you have passed the remnants of Buck Spring Lodge—George W. Vanderbilt's hunting cabin. Mount Pisgah is the most identifiable peak in Western North Carolina. On a clear day, the 339-foot television tower that crowns the mountain can be seen from seven surrounding counties. A hike to the base of the tower will reveal great views of Shining Rock Wilderness to the west and the French Broad River Basin to the east.

Route Details

Begin your hike to Mount Pisgah via Buck Spring Lodge at the Pisgah Inn off the Blue Ridge Parkway. Feel free to visit the snack bar and gift shop before you locate the trailhead at the north end of the parking lot. For a weather preview, check out their live webcam at pisgahinn.com.

Follow Buck Spring Trail uphill and into the woods. During late summer, several wildflowers, including joe-pye weed, pale blue asters, and field thistle, grow alongside one another.

At 0.7 mile into your hike, a trail junction leads to Little Bald summit. Continue straight on Buck Spring Trail to reach another nearby intersection with Laurel Mountain Trail. After bypassing Laurel Mountain Trail, stay vigilant and start looking to the right of the trail to spot the historic and often-hidden remains of Buck Spring Lodge.

George W. Vanderbilt (1862–1914) is arguably the most well-known, influential, and extravagant former resident of Western North Carolina. His Biltmore House, fashioned after a French chateau, has 250 rooms and is still recognized as the largest home in America. However, when Vanderbilt longed for a simpler resting place, he would travel 22 miles by horseback on the Shut-In Ridge Trail to his hunting cabin.

Though small compared with the Biltmore House, Buck Spring Lodge was hardly a rustic retreat. Built in 1895 by the same architects who designed the Biltmore House, Buck Spring Lodge featured hot and cold running water and electricity. The Biltmore Estate Archives suggest that there was a year-round caretaker and seasonal staff stationed at the lodge to serve the Vanderbilts and maintain the facilities. Along with the main lodge, the site also boasted a separate honeymoon cottage, garage, stable, kitchen/dining area, and playhouse for Vanderbilt's daughter, Cornelia.

Mount Pisgah via Buck Spring Lodge

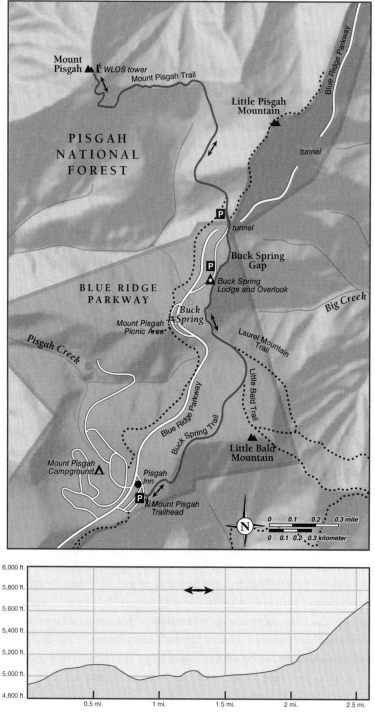

Knowing how large and grand this hunting cabin must have been, it is hard to believe that an uninformed hiker could miss it completely. But sadly, after George's wife, Edith, died in 1957, the Buck Spring property was sold to the National Park Service for the creation of the Blue Ridge Parkway, and the lodge was dismantled. Today, the foundations of the lodge and outer buildings are overgrown with weeds and rhododendron thickets. If it were not for the solitary informational sign beside the trail, most people would never know the significant history of this spot.

Beneath the site of Buck Spring Lodge, you will follow the path as it exits the woods and crosses a paved parkway overlook at Buck Spring Gap. To the east of the overlook, the trail reenters the woods for a quick 0.2-mile jaunt on the Mountains-to-Sea Trail (MST). This short section of the MST crosses the parkway unnoticeably as it winds through the woods above the Buck Spring tunnel and then descends to the Mount Pisgah parking lot.

The Mount Pisgah trailhead begins east of the parking lot. Just beyond the trailhead, a short spur trail leads to the Mount Pisgah campground and picnic area, but you should ignore this side trail and continue up the mountain. The beginning of the climb is relatively gentle. During summer, jewelweed and wild sunflowers line the trail, and a thick canopy of oak and poplar leaves provides shade from the sun.

At 2 miles the ascent becomes more difficult, and the last quarter mile to the summit is a heart-pounding crawl. Thankfully, when you reach the top, a terrific view of the surrounding mountains rewards all of your hard work. In fact, Mount Pisgah was named by Reverend George Newton in the early 18th century after the biblical Mount Pisgah, where Moses viewed the promised land for the first time.

You may be disappointed that a looming tower obscures the northern vista; if so, you are not the only one. The WLOS broadcast tower was built in 1954 and since then has been a source of controversy in Western North Carolina. Many people believe the tower should be removed from the top of the mountain. However, as long as the fixture remains on the mountain, it will make Pisgah the most easily recognizable peak in the Asheville area. It will also help provide a sense of perspective and distance as you climb to the top of other mountains.

After enjoying the view, hike back down Mount Pisgah and past Buck Spring Lodge to the trailhead.

Nearby Attractions

The Pisgah Inn, located near the trailhead, offers a restaurant, snack bar, and gift shop. Enjoy a meal with a view, overnight accommodations, and quick access to some of the best hikes in Pisgah National Forest.

Directions

Take the Blue Ridge Parkway south from Asheville for approximately 15 miles. The Pisgah Inn and trailhead parking lot are located on the left between mile markers 408 and 409.

A 339-FOOT BROADCASTING TOWER CROWNS MOUNT PISGAH.

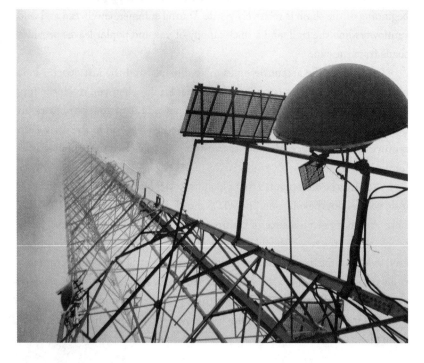

Pink Beds Loop

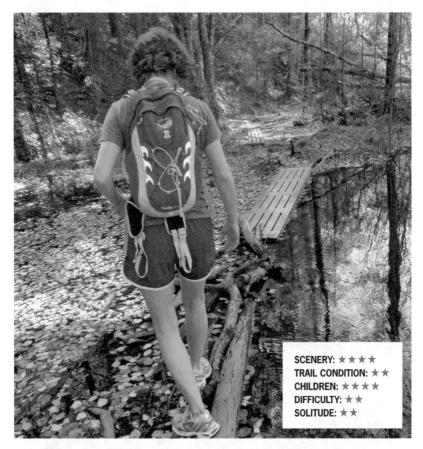

SCENERY: ★★★★
TRAIL CONDITION: ★★
CHILDREN: ★★★★
DIFFICULTY: ★★
SOLITUDE: ★★

IF IT HAS RAINED RECENTLY, YOU MAY NEED TO NAVIGATE WET SECTIONS OF THE PINK BEDS LOOP.

TRAILHEAD GPS COORDINATES: 35.353400, -82.778933

DISTANCE & CONFIGURATION: 5.4-mile loop

HIKING TIME: 3 hours

HIGHLIGHTS: The rare swamp pink lily

ELEVATION: 3,314' at trailhead, 3,170' at South Fork of Mills River

ACCESS: Free and always open

MAPS: National Geographic #780 *Pisgah Ranger District;* USGS *Shining Rock*

FACILITIES: Restrooms and a picnic pavilion in an open field east of the parking lot

WHEELCHAIR ACCESS: None

CONTACTS: Pisgah National Forest, Pisgah Ranger District, 828-877-3265, fs.usda.gov/nfsnc

Pink Beds Loop

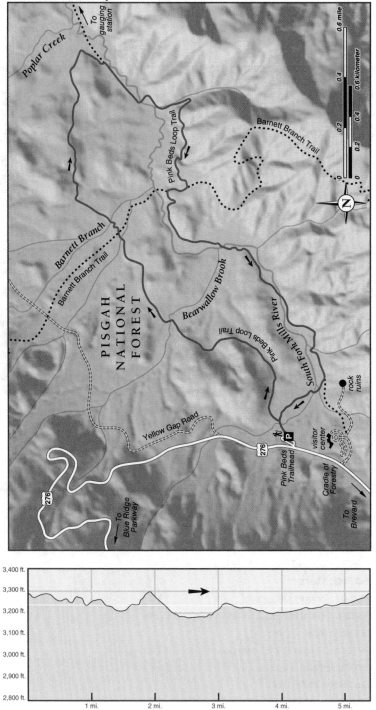

Overview

The Pink Beds Loop offers a fun and varied hike that travels through hardwood forests, on the edge of open fields, and beside peaceful streams. The final quarter of the hike passes through the pink bed wetlands and offers hikers the chance to catch a glimpse of the rare swamp pink lily. At times, the wetlands are impassable due to high water, but the alternate route still makes for a lovely day spent in the woods. The pavilion located near the trailhead makes this hike a popular destination for groups looking to picnic, hike, and perhaps throw Frisbees or play games in the open field near the start of the trail.

Route Details

The Pink Beds Loop will take you on a relatively level hike through the forests of Pink Beds Valley and beside formerly farmed open fields. On your hike you will intersect some of the waterways streaming through the Pink Beds. These water sources make Pink Beds a very fertile and lush valley, but they also can create some muddy hiking. In the past, beaver activity has flooded portions of the Pink Beds Loop. If the weather has been relatively dry, it is possible to navigate the wetlands on plank walkways, constructed and improvised bridges, without getting your feet wet. However, if it has rained within the past week, or if you are not inclined to balance on logs and hug onto trees, an alternate route on Barnett Branch Trail is recommended.

To begin your hike at Pink Beds, travel to the north end of the parking lot, where a faded wooden sign marks the beginning of the Pink Beds Loop. Travel 100 feet into the forest to where the trail splits. Veer left to hike the loop in a clockwise direction.

For the first mile of the hike, you will wander in and out of open fields. Today, the Forest Service maintains these open meadows to provide areas for wildlife, such as deer and wild turkeys, to feed. However, the European farmers who settled in the Pink Beds Valley once used these exposed tracts to raise crops and graze livestock. The land there was fertile and lush. However, a convenient trading market was not readily available, and the Pink Bed farmers had to transport their harvest to markets in Greenville, South Carolina, and even Charleston, South Carolina.

At 1.4 miles you will intersect Barnett Branch Trail. At this juncture you will want to continue hiking straight on the Pink Beds Loop; if you decide later on that you do not wish to explore the Pink Beds wetlands, then you will return to this same intersection toward the end of the hike.

Beyond the trail intersection, the path will lead you through rhododendron and mountain laurel thickets. Many locals believe that Pink Beds derived its name from the copious pink-and-white blooms on the mountain laurel trees and the bright-pink rhododendron flowers. However, a sign at the trailhead kiosk suggests that the flowering shrubs were only part of the reason the area became known as Pink Beds.

Centuries ago, Englishmen referred to all wildflowers as "pink," and the name "Pink Beds" could suggest that the area was filled with wildflowers of all different colors. Another theory suggests that the creeping pink phlox that once grew prominently in the valley was the source of the name. Regardless of which explanation is true, it is quite clear that for the past 200 years, the Pink Beds Valley has been filled with an array of beautiful wildflowers and continues to be to this day.

After hiking 2.4 miles, you will come to another trail intersection. This time the trail to the left leads to a nearby gauging station and trailhead off Forest Road 476, but you will want to continue right on the Pink Beds Loop. This begins the second half of the hike near the South Fork Mills River. Traveling close to the water, you will notice doghobble lining the creek and ferns overtaking the path. The trees that shade the water include oak, poplar, and short-needle pine trees.

When you arrive at the path's second intersection with Barnett Branch Trail at 3.6 miles, you will need to make a decision. If you want to keep dry feet and walk on a defined path, turn right on Barnett Branch Trail. Follow it back to the first intersection with the Pink Beds Loop, and then turn left to return to the trailhead on a balloon hike. If you want to have an adventure, potentially get muddy, view beaver habitats, and catch a glimpse of the rare swamp pink lily, continue straight on the Pink Beds Loop.

The main route now enters the Pink Beds wetlands area. This high-elevation mountain bog is home to the fire swamp lily. Pink Beds supports the second-highest population of this plant in the world, after the Pine Barrens of New Jersey. The best time to view the pink flower cluster that rises above the lily pad is in early spring.

If you've chosen to follow the Pink Beds Loop to completion, then you can try to keep your feet dry by walking on logs, hugging onto trees, and leaping from rock to rock. Or you can simply take off your shoes and embrace the cold, wet mud that fills the marsh. Whichever method you choose, you will navigate a route more similar to an obstacle course than a hiking path. When you arrive back at the trailhead, after wading for 1.6 miles, you will most likely have twigs in your hair, mud on your ankles, and a huge smile on your face.

Nearby Attractions

The Cradle of Forestry, birthplace of forestry in North America, lies just south of Pink Beds on US 276. The historic site offers interpretive trails, a visitor center, and a gift shop. The Cradle of Forestry is open Wednesday–Sunday 10 a.m.–5 p.m., from mid-April to mid-November. There is a modest entrance fee for visitors.

Directions

Take the Blue Ridge Parkway south from Asheville approximately 18 miles to mile marker 411. Look for US 276 and signs for the Cradle of Forestry. Turn south on US 276 and drive 3.5 miles. The Pink Beds picnic area and trailhead will be on your left. If you reach the Cradle of Forestry, you have gone too far.

From Brevard, take US 276 north 11.5 miles, past Looking Glass Falls and Sliding Rock. The Pink Beds entrance will be on your right, just past the Cradle of Forestry.

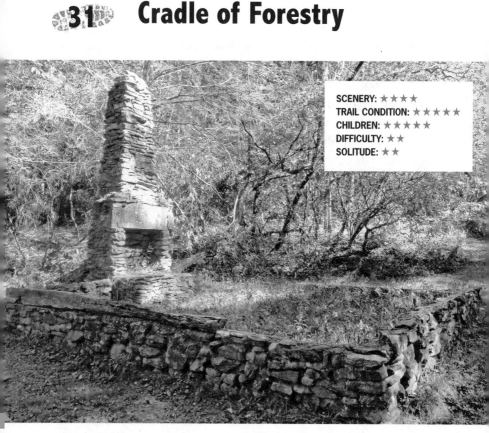

SCENERY: ★★★★
TRAIL CONDITION: ★★★★★
CHILDREN: ★★★★★
DIFFICULTY: ★★
SOLITUDE: ★★

THE FOUNDATION OF AN OLD HOMESTEAD ON THE FOREST FESTIVAL TRAIL

TRAILHEAD GPS COORDINATES: 35.350833, -82.779000

DISTANCE & CONFIGURATION: 2.2-mile figure eight

HIKING TIME: 1.5 hours

HIGHLIGHTS: The first school of forestry in North America

ELEVATION: 3,292' at trailhead, 3,262' at the tunnel underneath US 276

ACCESS: The Cradle of Forestry historic site is open Wednesday–Sunday 10 a.m.–5 p.m., mid-April–mid-November, and charges a modest entrance fee.

MAPS: National Geographic #780 *Pisgah Ranger District;* USGS *Shining Rock*

WHEELCHAIR ACCESS: Yes, at the visitor center and on the hiking trails

FACILITIES: Visitor center, museum, gift shop, and restrooms

COMMENTS: The Cradle of Forestry is a great place to take groups of children. Contact the office for group rates, educational programs, and scheduling.

CONTACTS: Cradle of Forestry: 828-877-3130, cradleofforestry.com; Pisgah National Forest, 828-257-4200, fs.usda.gov/nfsnc

Overview

The Cradle of Forestry is home to the first forestry school in North America and offers two interpretive trails. This hike combines both paths into a 2.2-mile figure eight. The first path, the Forest Festival Trail, teaches hikers about the plants and animals that define the surrounding habitat. The adjoining path, the Biltmore Campus Trail, takes you through the restored and reconstructed buildings that comprised the first forestry school in North America.

Route Details

Pink Beds Valley and the Cradle of Forestry is a region rich in history, biodiversity, and recreational opportunities. Inhabited since the early 1800s, the lush and level tract of land, below the slopes of Mount Pisgah, was first a rural farming community. In 1889, George W. Vanderbilt bought the property to be a part of his Biltmore Estate and appointed Gifford Pinchot to manage the land. Pinchot later left to become the first chief of the Forest Service.

German forester Dr. Carl Schenck succeeded Pinchot at the Biltmore Estate. Schenck used a portion of the Pink Beds Valley to form the first forestry school in the United States, the Cradle of Forestry. Schenck worked diligently to restore the surrounding forests to health after years of careless logging and farming. Upon George Vanderbilt's death in 1914 his wife Edith, sold 87,000 acres of forestland, including Pink Beds Valley and the Cradle of Forestry, to the Forest Service.

In 1968, the Cradle of Forestry was designated as a National Historic Site, and today the facility delights young and old with a state-of-the-art visitor center and two wheelchair-accessible interpretive trails. The hike on this significant plot of land starts behind the visitor center and first heads east to explore the Forest Festival Trail.

Before reaching the start of the Forest Festival Trail, you will pass a unique tree on your left. Stuart Roosa, a revered American astronaut, had a special connection to this tree. Roosa traveled with the seed for this four-decades-old sycamore tree on a journey into outer space. In fact, Roosa, a former smoke jumper for the Forest Service, took 500 seeds with him on an expedition that orbited the moon. Then, upon his return to Earth, he presented the seeds as a gift to the Forest Service.

Cradle of Forestry

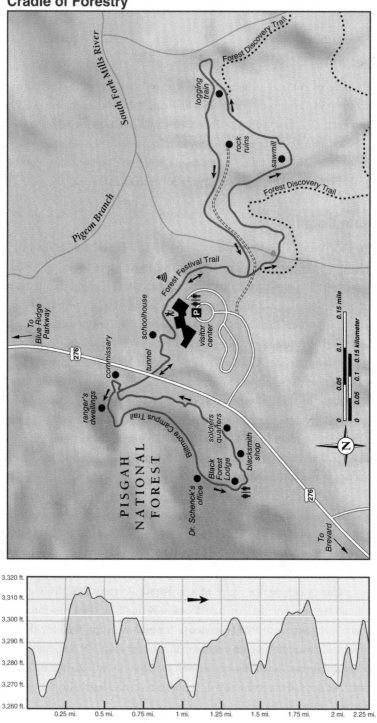

Continuing past the "out of this world" sycamore tree, you will arrive at the start of the Forest Festival Trail. Veer right (south) to hike the trail counterclockwise.

During the age of the Biltmore Forestry School, Schenck would hold an annual Forest Festival and invite leading individuals in the lumber industry, politicians, and media members. The celebration at the forestry school allowed Schenck to relay advances in discoveries in the world of forestry.

The informative Forest Festival Trail will lead you on a self-guided tour of some of the innovations and experiments at the Cradle of Forestry. From a seedling garden to a sawmill, and from the rock foundations of a homestead to the remnants of a fish hatchery, the path and informational placards guide you on a tour of an outdoor museum that informs you about different types of trees, animals, and forestry practices. For many, the highlight of the Forest Festival Trail is the Climax train engine and steam log loader, located on a reconstructed narrow-gauge rail. The train and log loader were important tools used to deliver the lumber from the forest to the towns, mills, and markets in the valley.

At the conclusion of the Forest Festival loop, return on the paved path to the back side of the visitor center, and then continue hiking west to explore the neighboring Biltmore Campus Trail. Just as the Forest Festival Trail gives insight into the practices of early forestry, the Biltmore Campus Trail provides a glimpse of what life was like for the foresters who cared for these natural resources.

The Biltmore Campus Trail's first stop is at the restored schoolhouse, where forestry students would spend the morning learning from textbooks before venturing out in the afternoon for hands-on experience. After leaving the one-room schoolhouse, the path travels through a tunnel under US 276 and arrives at the living quarters and commissary. The primitive conditions will make you appreciate how hardy the year-round forestry students and members of this mountain community must have been, especially in winter.

As you continue on the path, you will reach additional living quarters, a toolshed, a garden, and Dr. Schenck's office. It is always humbling for locals to think that not only was the practice of American forestry first cultivated at the Biltmore school, but two of the biggest names in this field, Pinchot and Schenck, also spent significant time in these mountains and woods right outside of Asheville.

After retracing your steps to the back side of the visitor center, the hike and your outside museum visit will conclude; but before you leave, be sure to go in and tour the interactive exhibits and videos. It is likely that upon leaving the historic site you will feel differently about the trees and forest that surround the entrance than when you first arrived.

Directions

From Asheville, take the Blue Ridge Parkway south and travel approximately 18 miles to mile marker 411. Look for US 276 and signs for the Cradle of Forestry. Turn south on US 276 and drive 4 miles. The Cradle of Forestry will be just past Pink Beds on your left.

From Brevard, take US 276 north 11 miles, past Looking Glass Falls and Sliding Rock. The Cradle of Forestry entrance will be on your right. If you reach the Pink Beds parking area, you have gone too far.

THIS LODGE WAS ORIGINALLY CONSTRUCTED TO HOUSE RANGERS IN BILTMORE FOREST.

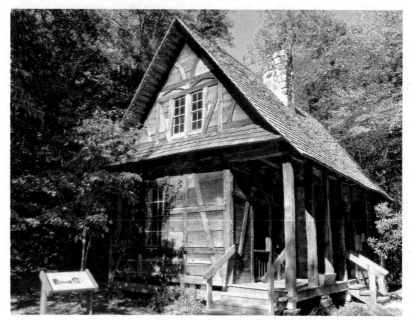

32 Shining Rock

SCENERY: ★ ★ ★ ★ ★
TRAIL CONDITION: ★ ★
CHILDREN: ★
DIFFICULTY: ★ ★ ★ ★ ★
SOLITUDE: ★ ★

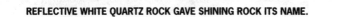

REFLECTIVE WHITE QUARTZ ROCK GAVE SHINING ROCK ITS NAME.

TRAILHEAD GPS COORDINATES: 35.365950, -82.818317

DISTANCE & CONFIGURATION: 8.5-mile loop

HIKING TIME: 7 hours

HIGHLIGHTS: Great views from the large quartz deposit known as Shining Rock and substantial creekside walking

ELEVATION: 3,354' at trailhead, 5,957' at Shining Rock

ACCESS: Free and always open

MAPS: National Geographic #780 *Pisgah Ranger District;* USGS *Shining Rock, Cruso*

FACILITIES: None

WHEELCHAIR ACCESS: None

COMMENTS: This is a very difficult hike. Leave early in the morning to allow for plenty of daylight to complete this loop.

CONTACTS: Pisgah National Forest, Pisgah Ranger District, 828-877-3265, fs.usda.gov/nfsnc

Shining Rock

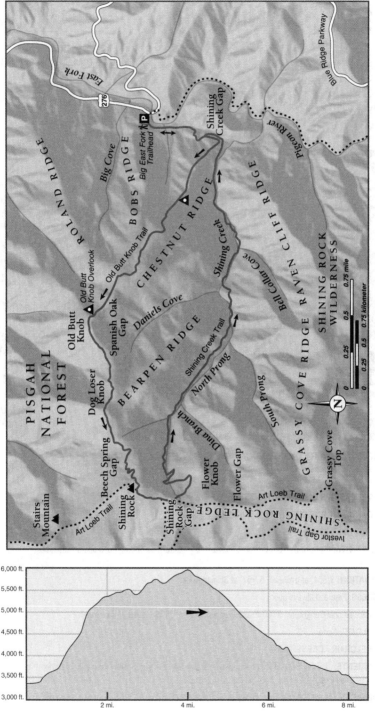

Overview

The hike to Shining Rock from Big East Fork Trailhead is very difficult. By taking Old Butt Knob Trail to the summit, you will gain more than 2,500 feet in 4 miles. However, the views from the large quartz garden at Shining Rock make the strenuous effort worthwhile. When you are ready to return to the base of the mountain, you will take the scenic Shining Creek Trail. This route parallels a cascading mountain stream until it meets the Big East Fork River near the trailhead.

Route Details

Begin the hike at the Big East Fork Trailhead off US 276. Often on weekends the parking area at the trailhead is full, in which case there is an open field on the east side of US 276 that accommodates overflow parking. The start of Shining Creek Trail is located at the west end of the parking lot, and it parallels the north bank of the Big East Fork River into the woods. Because this trail falls within the Shining Rock Creek Wilderness, none of the trails are marked. You will need to pay extra-close attention to the hiking directions and should definitely bring a map and compass.

After 0.2 mile the trail veers away from the river and starts climbing gradually through a hardwood forest of maple, birch, hickory, and Fraser magnolia trees. At 0.7 mile you will hike into a small dip and then rise to the crest of the next climb. This apex is where you leave Shining Creek Trail and turn northwest onto Old Butt Knob Trail. Again, it is easy to miss this turnoff, so be extra vigilant and look to your right for the trail that seemingly veers straight up the mountainside.

The first segment of Old Butt Knob Trail will leave you instantly fatigued—head hanging, chest heaving, and feeling like an old butt. The trail travels a strenuous grade up the spine of Chestnut Ridge, and you can sense the slight variations in how steep the trail is by the burning sensation in your calf muscles.

After 0.3 mile of crawling up Old Butt Knob Trail, the path briefly levels off before once again angling upward. At 1.2 miles look for a rocky overlook on the left. This is a great place to take a well-deserved rest. The beautiful views of Daniels Cove and Bear Pen Ridge are a nice reward for all your hard effort. The scenery will also motivate you to keep moving up the mountain and discover the other great overlooks still to come.

Just past the 1.5-mile mark, you will come across something perhaps even more beautiful than a mountain view—a switchback. The brief contouring zigzag is a sign that the hardest part of the climb is over, and even though the trail continues to take a direct route up the mountain, the steepest pitch is behind you.

The forest around you will begin to transition from a canopy of maple, oak, and beech trees to a wilderness dotted with dark-green spruce and fir trees. At 2.4 miles you will reach Old Butt Knob, where a rocky outcrop provides extensive panoramas of Shining Rock Wilderness. On a clear day, you can even spot the gleam of the quartz rock that awaits you on top of Shining Rock ledge. In fact, Shining Rock earned its name from the reflective nature of the quartz outcrops that line the ridge.

A LOOK SOUTHWEST FROM SHINING ROCK INTO THE SHINING ROCK AND MIDDLE PRONG WILDERNESSES

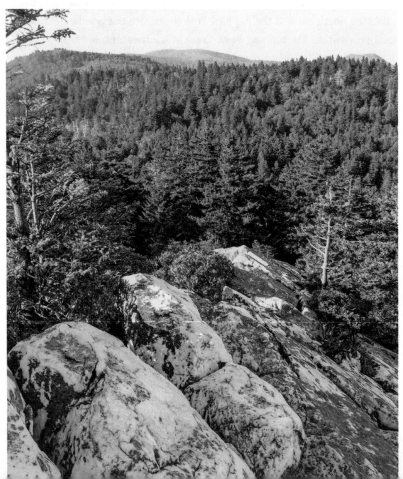

Past Old Butt Knob, you will make a moderate ascent up Dog Loser Knob. Then you will enjoy a relatively flat hike that leads to your last uphill push to the top of Shining Rock. Old Butt Knob Trail hits the ridgeline just to the north of Shining Rock. There is a spur trail on the ridge that leads to the west, but you will want to turn south and hike downhill.

The next 0.2 mile offers several spur trails that lead to different parts of Shining Rock. Feel free to explore these small detours and then find a spot on the bright-white quartz rock that defines Shining Rock to take in the view and enjoy a well-deserved snack. Most of the perches on top of Shining Rock, where people stop to rest, reveal views of Pisgah Ridge, Tennent Mountain, and the Middle Prong Wilderness.

When you are ready to leave Shining Rock and start your journey down the mountain, continue south along the ridge, ignoring multiple rabbit trails that lead to nearby campsites. You will come into a small grassy opening at Shining Rock Gap. There is a trail that veers off to the west, but you will want to bear left and continue hiking south. Within a few hundred feet, you will come to another trail junction. This time a path to the east will lead off the ridge and plunge downhill. Turn left here onto Shining Creek Trail.

The first part of this trail can be slick and wet, but soon the terrain channels the seeping water sources near the top of the mountain, and within 0.2 mile you will be hiking next to a well-defined creek. The path follows the creek for the next 3 miles and reveals several small cascades on its journey down the mountain. After traveling a cumulative 7.5 miles, you will veer north away from the creek. One mile later you will arrive back at your car in the Big East Fork parking area.

Directions

From Asheville, drive approximately 20 miles on the Blue Ridge Parkway to milepost 411. Before you reach milepost 412, turn north on US 276 and travel 2.8 miles. The Big East Fork Trailhead will be on your left.

From Canton, take NC 215 south 5.3 miles and then turn left onto Market Street. Stay on Market Street 0.3 mile and then turn left onto US 276, heading south. Travel 12 miles on US 276. Big East Fork Trailhead will be on your right.

Black Balsam Knob High Loop

SCENERY: ★ ★ ★ ★ ★
TRAIL CONDITION: ★ ★ ★
CHILDREN: ★ ★ ★
DIFFICULTY: ★ ★ ★
SOLITUDE: ★ ★ ★

A VIEW DOWN YELLOWSTONE PRONG FROM THE SLOPES OF BLACK BALSAM KNOB

TRAILHEAD GPS COORDINATES: 35.325797, -82.881964

DISTANCE & CONFIGURATION: 5.2-mile loop

HIKING TIME: 3.5 hours

HIGHLIGHTS: Panoramic views from Tennent Mountain and Black Balsam Knob

ELEVATION: 5,818' at trailhead, 6,205' at Black Balsam Knob

ACCESS: Free and always open, but vehicle access to this hike is unavailable when the Blue Ridge Parkway is closed. Check nps.gov/blri for real-time road closures.

MAPS: National Geographic #780 *Pisgah Ranger District;* USGS *Shining Rock, Sam Knob*

FACILITIES: Pit toilets at the Black Balsam Knob parking area

WHEELCHAIR ACCESS: None

COMMENTS: Several unmarked side trails lead from Black Balsam ridge; use a USGS or National Geographic map to follow them. Also, because of the high elevation and lack of tree cover, carrying sunscreen is advisable year-round.

CONTACTS: Blue Ridge Parkway, 828-298-0398, nps.gov/blri; Shining Rock Wilderness, 828-257-4200, fs.usda.gov/nfsnc

Overview

Black Balsam Knob is a favorite destination of many Western North Carolina hikers. For sure, the views from there and from Tennent Mountain are some of the best in the Southeast. You will see for yourself on this loop hike: it follows the Ivestor Gap Trail—a former road—to the Shining Rock Wilderness boundary and then loops back to the parking lot on the most dramatic and scenic section of the Art Loeb Trail.

Route Details

In Asheville, when Black Balsam comes up in conversation, the topic is usually followed by stories of a romantic first kiss, a wedding proposal, a fun-filled afternoon of blueberry picking with friends, or a quiet evening spent watching the sunset over the Blue Ridge Mountains. This area is truly magical and a special spot for many local residents.

This hike begins from the Black Balsam Knob parking area at the end of Black Balsam Knob Road. Start by heading for the Ivestor Gap Trailhead at the north end of the parking lot. For most of the year, this narrow dirt road is closed to vehicular traffic, but in fall and early winter it opens to four-wheel-drive cars and trucks. During this period, hikers should be cautious of oncoming traffic.

For some background on your adventure, it's interesting to know that the level terrain of the Ivestor Gap Trail was initially created as a railroad bed for a logging operation. At the turn of the 20th century, the Champion Fiber Company bought large tracts of land in the Pisgah and Shining Rock area for harvesting pulpwood for the paper mill in Canton. This endeavor decimated the mountain slopes of chestnut, oak, hemlock, Fraser fir, and spruce trees. Then, in 1925, a huge wildfire destroyed the railroads, the remaining trees, and important soil nutrients.

As a result, the surrounding terrain was left barren and forgotten. In 1934, the Forest Service purchased the land, and the terrain has been slowly regenerating since that time. Even though nine decades have passed since the area was ravished by logging and wildfire, there are still only patches of spruce trees where dense spruce forests once thrived.

As you travel along the Ivestor Gap Trail, enjoy terrific views of Sam Knob and the Middle Prong Wilderness to your left (west). After 1.9 miles the

Black Balsam Knob High Loop

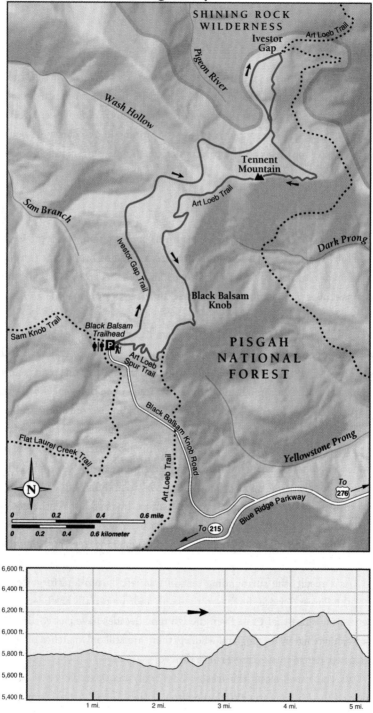

old railroad bed briefly comes in contact with the Art Loeb Trail. If you wish to shorten the hike by nearly a mile, you can turn right and join the Art Loeb at this point; however, the recommended route follows the Ivestor Gap Trail another 0.4 mile to the wooden sign that marks the start of the Shining Rock Wilderness. You will need to pay special attention at the Shining Rock boundary to turn hard right (south) onto the Art Loeb Trail and follow it due south, up a neighboring hillside.

Once on the Art Loeb Trail, you wind up the ridge to Tennent Mountain. Its namesake, Asheville resident Dr. Gaillard Stoney Tennent, was the first president of the Carolina Mountain Club. The Tennent Mountain summit reveals a 360-degree view of the surrounding Blue Ridge Mountains. At this point, you can look east and see the Asheville city limits, with the Black Mountain range in the background. You can also look west and make out the faint ridges of Great Smoky Mountains National Park. Wow!

From Tennent Mountain, continue on the Art Loeb Trail through a patch of blueberry bushes and Apiaceae plants to the neighboring gap. Veer right to stay on the Art Loeb Trail and begin a gradual uphill climb to Black Balsam Knob. When you arrive at the knob, another amazing panoramic view of the Blue Ridge rewards you. The vista is similar to that atop Tennent Mountain, but this one also has a rock outcrop that offers a great place to sit and study the southern reaches of Pisgah National Forest, including Looking Glass Rock.

From Black Balsam Knob, hike south down a rocky eroded trail into a neighboring notch. Then travel the spine of the ridge to the final high point of the trail. Because of the proximity to the trailhead, there are several crisscrossing rabbit trails that intersect the path. Some of these unmarked trails lead to berry thickets, and others go to campsites. To remain on the Art Loeb Trail, stay along the backbone of the ridge.

At the top of the next high point, you will arrive at a trail junction with the Art Loeb Spur Trail. Take one last moment to look around and enjoy the view before descending the spur trail to your right. This 0.5-mile path provides one of the only sections of the hike with tree cover: a canopy of rhododendron, mountain laurel, and ash. This vivid green tunnel will lead you off the mountain and back to the Black Balsam Knob parking area to conclude your hike.

Directions

From Asheville, take the Blue Ridge Parkway south toward Mount Pisgah. Drive past Mount Pisgah and Graveyard Fields to mile marker 420, then turn right onto Black Balsam Knob Road/Forest Road 816. Follow the road 1.2 miles to the Black Balsam Knob parking lot, information kiosk, and trailhead.

THE ART LOEB TRAIL LEADS TO THE TOP OF BLACK BALSAM KNOB.

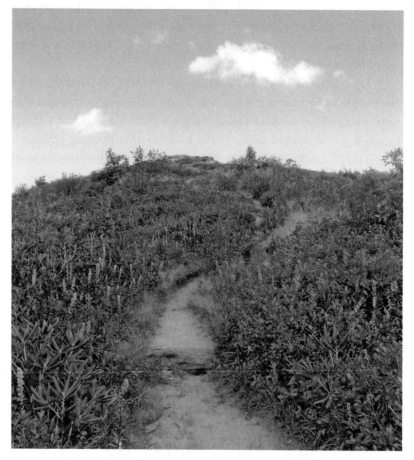

Sam Knob

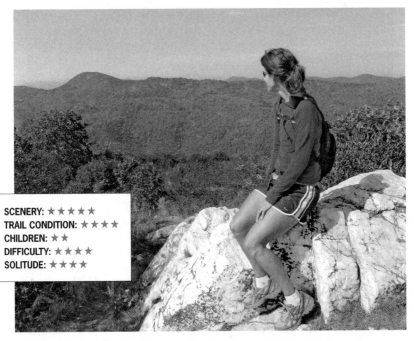

LOOKING DOWN ON THE FLAT LAUREL CREEK VALLEY FROM AN OUTCROP

TRAILHEAD GPS COORDINATES: 35.325850, -82.882017

DISTANCE & CONFIGURATION: 9.6-mile loop

HIKING TIME: 5 hours

HIGHLIGHTS: Extensive views from Sam Knob Trail and Summit Trail, creekside walking, and mountain laurel tunnels

ELEVATION: 5,823' at trailhead, 6,073' at Sam Knob's summit

ACCESS: Free and always open, but vehicle access to this hike is unavailable when the Blue Ridge Parkway is closed. Check nps.gov/blri for real-time road closures.

MAPS: National Geographic #780 *Pisgah Ranger District;* USGS *Sam Knob*

FACILITIES: Pit toilets at the trailhead

WHEELCHAIR ACCESS: None

COMMENTS: This hike has many variations and shorter options. Bring along a trail map if you wish to find a different or quicker route back to the parking area.

CONTACTS: Blue Ridge Parkway, 828-298-0398, nps.gov/blri; Pisgah National Forest, 828-257-4200, fs.usda.gov/nfsnc

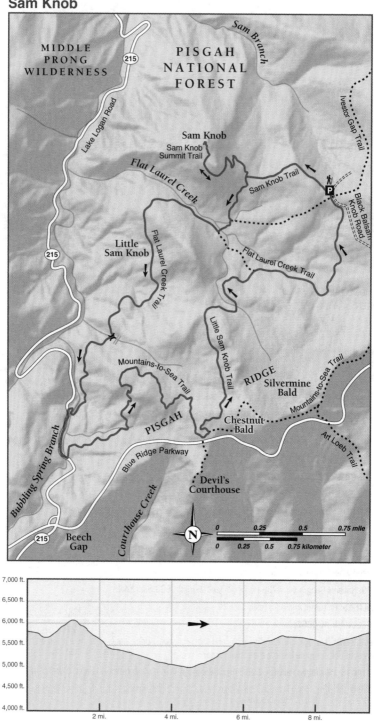

Overview

This hike follows the Sam Knob Trail through an open meadow to the Sam Knob Summit Trail, where a short out-and-back provides terrific views of Black Balsam and Devil's Courthouse. The route then takes Flat Laurel Creek Trail and parallels the flowing water to NC 215. After a short road walk, the hike dives back into a hardwood forest on the Mountains-to-Sea Trail (MST). The path then skirts the south side of Little Sam Knob before connecting back to the trailhead on the Little Sam Knob and Flat Laurel Creek Trails.

Route Details

The trailhead for this hike is behind the pit toilets in the Black Balsam Knob parking area. Follow the dirt path behind the latrines for about 100 yards and then veer right (northwest) onto the Sam Knob Trail. Follow the path through a youngish forest of maple, beech, and mountain laurel trees.

After 0.3 mile you will exit the forest at a large open meadow. Continue through the grassy field toward Sam Knob and pass beside seasonal wildflowers such as white yarrow, purple asters, and white wood asters. At 0.6 mile you will come to the start of the Sam Knob Summit Trail. Turn right on this 0.7-mile spur trail and hike the gradual ascent to the top of Sam Knob, where terrific vistas of Shining Rock Wilderness and Middle Prong Wilderness extend west and north. The Blue Ridge Parkway and Pisgah Ridge rise to your south.

This terrain was not spared from the same raging wildfire that burned across Graveyard Fields and Shining Rock Wilderness. You will notice the shrub-filled heath areas surrounding Sam Knob that are still recovering from the ravaging effects of both the logging and wildfires that plagued the region during the first half of the 20th century.

From this viewpoint, you can also look south on the jagged slope of Devil's Courthouse. Devil's Courthouse gets its name from a Cherokee legend that claims an evil spirit, who passes judgment on individuals lacking courage, lives within this mountain. Between Sam Knob and Devil's Courthouse, you will spot the two-toned slopes of Little Sam Knob. The south slope of the mountain was allowed to reforest naturally and is covered in light-green hardwood trees and shrubs; however, the north slope was replanted with dark-green spruce trees after the logging operation ceased.

After savoring the views at the summit, backtrack down the Sam Knob Summit Trail to the Sam Knob Trail, and then follow it south toward Flat Laurel Creek. You will pass several backcountry campsites prior to reaching the creek at 2.5 miles. (*Note:* Backcountry campers are required to use bearproof canisters in this area.) Cross the stream and turn right on Flat Laurel Creek Trail. This path follows an old railroad bed next to the creek. The narrow-gauge railroad was once used to transport lumber down the mountain to Sunburst in the West Fork Pigeon River Valley. The route passes several small cascades, and at 4 miles it crosses the creek on a cement bridge that displays a tall waterfall to the left.

The Flat Laurel Creek Trail eventually dead-ends at NC 215. Turn left at the paved highway and complete a short 0.3-mile road walk to meet the Mountains-to-Sea Trail (MST). Directly after crossing over a bridge, turn left on the white-blazed MST and follow it on a gradual ascent through a long green tunnel of rhododendrons. The trail contours a small stream and crosses the skinny waterway on a log bridge. There, you will leave behind the rhododendron thickets and enter a spruce forest. Eventually, the trail opens up into a hemlock grove where the path becomes lost amid a carpet of hemlock needles. Be careful to follow the white circles through the planted grove and back into the forest.

At 6.9 miles you will reach a blue-blazed trail that leads right to Devil's Courthouse. Veer left and remain on the MST another 0.4 mile to a junction with Little Sam Knob Trail. Turn left onto Little Sam Knob Trail; in about 100 yards, you will need to leap across a small stream. The trail then contours beneath the southeast slope of Little Sam Knob before it terminates at the Flat Laurel Creek Trail.

Turn right onto Flat Laurel Creek Trail to complete your loop. On your journey back to the trailhead you will enjoy some of the same expansive views that you relished on the first section of the hike, except you will be looking *at* Sams Knob instead of *from* Sams Knob. The pleasant railroad bed is lined with mountain ash trees and dotted with purple gentian flowers.

After hiking a total of 9.6 miles, Flat Laurel Creek Trail will reach the south end of the Black Balsam Knob parking area.

Directions

From Asheville, take the Blue Ridge Parkway south toward Mount Pisgah. Drive past Mount Pisgah and Graveyard Fields to mile marker 420, then turn right onto Black Balsam Knob Road/Forest Road 816. Follow the road 1.2 miles to the Black Balsam Knob parking lot, information kiosk, and trailhead. The Sam Knob Trailhead is located in the Black Balsam Knob parking area at the end of FR 816.

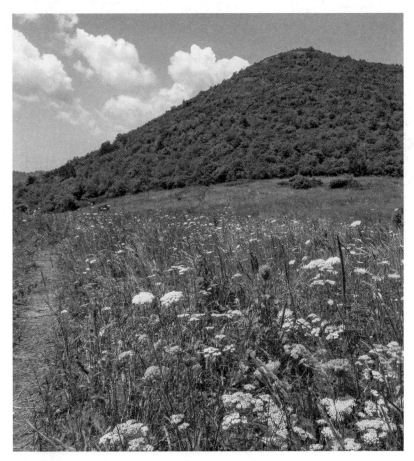

WILDFLOWERS CARPET THE MEADOW BELOW SAM KNOB.

Cold Mountain

SCENERY: ★ ★ ★ ★ ★
TRAIL CONDITION: ★ ★ ★
CHILDREN: ★
DIFFICULTY: ★ ★ ★ ★ ★
SOLITUDE: ★ ★

THE ART LOEB TRAIL PASSES THROUGH NORTH CAROLINA'S LARGEST WILDERNESS AREA, SHINING ROCK.

TRAILHEAD GPS COORDINATES: 35.387097, -82.895725

DISTANCE & CONFIGURATION: 10-mile out-and-back

HIKING TIME: 7.5 hours

HIGHLIGHTS: A beautiful, wooded walk to the summit of a famous literary peak, Cold Mountain

ELEVATION: 3,260' at trailhead, 6,005' on top of Cold Mountain

ACCESS: Free and always open

MAPS: National Geographic #780 *Pisgah Ranger District;* USGS *Cruso*

FACILITIES: None

WHEELCHAIR ACCESS: None

COMMENTS: Allow a full day to reach the summit of Cold Mountain. The trailhead is just over a 1-hour drive from Asheville, so 10 hours should be allotted for this hike door-to-door.

CONTACTS: Pisgah National Forest, Pisgah Ranger District, 828-877-3265, fs.usda.gov/nfsnc

Overview

When Charles Frazier's Civil War novel, *Cold Mountain*, came out in 1997 and subsequently sold more than 3 million copies, the wooded 6,000-foot mountain that casts its shadow just northwest of Asheville became known around the world. The out-and-back hike to the top of Cold Mountain starts just south of Camp Daniel Boone and climbs steadily uphill for 5 miles to the summit. Savor directionally limited but spectacular views from the summit and a beautiful mixed hardwood forest leading to the peak.

Route Details

National Book Award winner Charles Frazier was born in Asheville, North Carolina, and grew up in the Andrews and Franklin area of Western North Carolina. His first book, *Cold Mountain*, brought immediate attention to the spectacular mountain that dominates the landscape south of Canton. In his book, Frazier explores themes of humanity's relationship with nature, isolation, and self-discovery. If you decide to attempt the challenging 10-mile round-trip to the summit of Cold Mountain, then you will most likely relate to those same topics on your hike.

The trailhead for Cold Mountain is located on the south edge of Camp Daniel Boone, and the roads leading to the trailhead are circuitous and frequently change names. You should bring a street map, your smartphone, plus some tarot cards and a lucky rabbit's foot to augment the directions included in this guidebook. Actually, just type in 3647 Little East Fork Road, Canton, North Carolina, or the above coordinates on your smartphone, then go a little past the camp to the trailhead.

The Cold Mountain Trailhead also serves as the northern terminus of the Art Loeb Trail. To begin your hike, follow the Art Loeb Trail east and uphill. Thankfully, unlike most of the confusing trails and unmarked intersections in the Shining Rock Wilderness, the hike to the top of Cold Mountain is a generally straightforward, easy path to follow. The only trail junction will come once you reach the ridge.

If you are expecting spectacular mountain views leading up to Cold Mountain, then you will be disappointed. The first 3.5 miles of hiking lie entirely within the woods. That said, the dark and dense hardwood forest that lines the

Cold Mountain

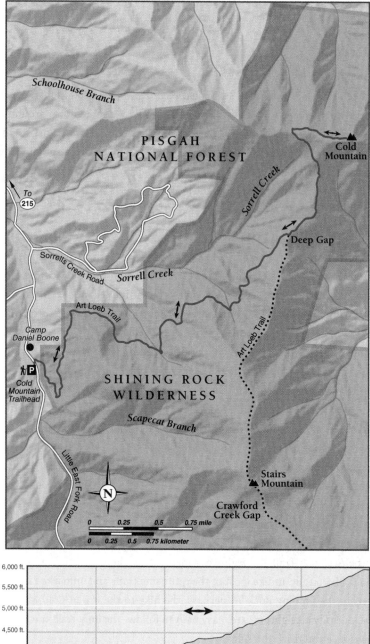

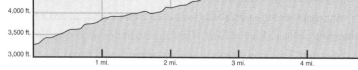

path is intimately beautiful and provides a sense of isolation and wilderness. The woods on the back side of Cold Mountain are very quiet, and you rarely will hear even a distant car or a plane flying overhead.

The first 1 mile of walking follows a steady uphill grade that will get your blood pumping and cause you to take off that extra top layer of clothing. After the first mile, the climb moderates and rocks litter the trail. Although this trail up Cold Mountain is indeed challenging and continues almost entirely uphill, the ascent is not as steep or difficult as trails, such as Old Butt Knob, that ascend the opposite slope. The Art Loeb Trail does a nice job of contouring the mountain and gaining elevation gradually.

At 1.8 miles you will cross a clear mountain brook, a tributary of Sorrell Creek. And after 3 miles the hike will increase in difficulty as you make a final 0.5-mile uphill push to reach Deep Gap. At Deep Gap you will find a small grassy opening. You may want to take a quick rest there and eat a snack before climbing the remaining 1.5 miles to the summit. When you are ready to leave Deep Gap, notice that several trails depart the grassy field. The Art Loeb Trail exits to the south, and several spur trails lead off the ridge to nearby camping spots. From the middle of the gap, make a 90-degree left turn and hike north on the spine of the ridge to follow the Cold Mountain Trail.

The ascent up Cold Mountain is much like the rest of the hike—densely wooded and uphill. At 4.4 miles, pass a piped spring that is a mere trickle during dry periods. Continuing past the water source, you will begin to pass several backcountry campsites. Some of these sites on the north side of the ridge offer views of the farmland below.

The final 0.1 mile of walking will reveal your best views of the hike: several rock outcrops near the summit provide gorgeous southern views of the Great Balsam Mountains. At 5 miles you will know you have arrived at the true summit of Cold Mountain when you spy the geological survey marker anchored in the rocks.

Congratulations! You are now above 6,000 feet on a summit that is world famous in modern literature. And now you have a gradual 5-mile descent to enjoy as you savor your accomplishment. As you head down, you no doubt will wonder why—with such natural beauty all around you—was the 2003 film *Cold Mountain,* starring Jude Law, Nicole Kidman, and Renée Zellweger, filmed in Romania and not in the true shadows of Cold Mountain?

Nearby Attractions

Camp Daniel Boone borders the Cold Mountain Trailhead. Enjoy viewing the scenic area as you drive through the main campus. The camp is an excellent way to initiate future adventurers into the great outdoors.

Directions

From Asheville, take I-40 west to exit 27, joining US 74 West for 3.1 miles. Turn right at exit 104 to join US 23 Business South for 2.2 miles, then veer left at the traffic circle onto Ratliff Cove. Follow Ratliff Cove for 0.4 mile, then keep straight as the road you are on becomes Raccoon Road. Follow Raccoon Road for 1.4 miles, then turn left onto US 276 South. After 2.8 miles, turn right on Edwards Cove Road. Follow Edwards Cove Road for 1.6 miles, then veer right onto Lake Logan Road. Follow Lake Logan Road for 3.1 miles, then take an acute left onto Little East Fork Road. Drive 3.7 miles to Camp Daniel Boone. Proceed through Camp Daniel Boone to reach a large gravel lot at the dead end of the public road (a private gated road continues beyond the trailhead).

Appendix A:
Outdoor Retailers

BLACK DOME MOUNTAIN SPORTS
blackdome.com
140 Tunnel Road
Asheville, NC 28805
800-678-2367

DIAMOND BRAND OUTDOORS
diamondbrandoutdoors.com
53 Biltmore Ave.
Asheville, NC 28801
828-771-4761

DICK'S SPORTING GOODS
dickssportinggoods.com
107 A River Hills Road
Asheville, NC 28805
828-299-0077

MAST GENERAL STORE
mastgeneralstore.com
15 Biltmore Ave.
Asheville, NC 28801
828-232-1883

527 N. Main St.
Hendersonville, NC 28792
828-696-1883

**NANTAHALA OUTDOOR
CENTER ASHEVILLE**
noc.com
290 Macon Ave.
Asheville, NC 28804
828-251-1615

REI
rei.com/stores/117
31 Schenck Pkwy.
Asheville, NC 28803
828-687-0918

**SECOND GEAR
(CONSIGNMENT SHOP)**
secondgearwnc.com
99 Riverside Dr.
Asheville, NC 28801
828-258-0757

TAKE A HIKE
takeahikenc.com
100 Sutton Ave.
Black Mountain, NC 28711
828-669-0811

Appendix B:
Hiking Clubs

You will never have to solo hike in Western North Carolina. This region is home to several very active hiking groups.

APPALACHIAN TRAIL CONSERVANCY (ATC), SOUTHERN OFFICE

appalachiantrail.org
160A Zillicoa St.
Asheville, NC 28801
828-254-3708

Join this group for hiking information, activities, and volunteer opportunities.

CAROLINA MOUNTAIN CLUB (CMC)

carolinamountainclub.org
P. O. Box 68
Asheville, NC 28802

The CMC is one of the country's premier hiking clubs. An annual membership fee gets you in. Members are invited to attend more than 175 events each year. Activities range from group hikes to trail-maintenance outings to club socials.

MOUNTAINS-TO-SEA TRAIL (MST)

mountainstosea.org
3509 Haworth Drive, Suite 210
Raleigh, NC 27609
919-825-0297

As with the ATC, above, the MST welcomes new members and offers volunteer opportunities.

Index

W

water, drinking, 9, 12
Waterfall Creek, 73
waterfalls, best hikes for, xi
weather, 8–9
west of Asheville
   described, 2
   featured hikes, 165–200
   map, 164
West Nile virus, 13
West Prong Hickey Fork, 47, 48

Wheelchair Access (hike profile), 7
whistle, 12
Whiteoak Flats Branch, 42
Wildcat Rock, 1, 117–121
Wildcat Rock Trail, 110
wildflowers, best hikes for, xi
wildlife, best hikes for, xi
Wilson, Tom, 95
WLOS broadcast tower, Mount Pisgah,
   169–170

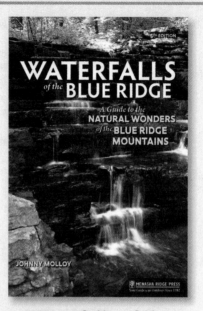

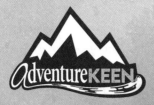

The Story of AdventureKEEN

We are an independent nature and outdoor activity publisher. Our founding dates back more than 40 years, guided then and now by our love of being in the woods and on the water, by our passion for reading and books, and by the sense of wonder and discovery made possible by spending time recreating outdoors in beautiful places.

It is our mission to share that wonder and fun with our readers, especially with those who haven't yet experienced all the physical and mental health benefits that nature and outdoor activity can bring.

In addition, we strive to teach about responsible recreation so that the natural resources and habitats we cherish and rely upon will be available for future generations.

We are a small team deeply rooted in the places where we live and work. We have been shaped by our communities of origin—primarily Birmingham, Alabama; Cincinnati, Ohio; and the northern suburbs of Minneapolis, Minnesota. Drawing on the decades of experience of our staff and our awareness of the industry, the marketplace, and the world at large, we have shaped a unique vision and mission for a company that serves our readers and authors.

We hope to meet you out on the trail someday.

#bewellbeoutdoors

About the Author

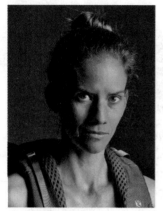

Photo: Keith Wright

JENNIFER PHARR DAVIS IS A LOVER OF LONG TRAILS and good stories. She has inspired women and men across the country with her message that "the trail is there for everyone at every phase of life" and has made a name for herself as a National Geographic Adventurer of the Year, hiker, speaker, and author. Jennifer set the overall fastest known time on the Appalachian Trail in 2011 by hiking 47 miles a day for 46 straight days. She was featured in the 2020 IMAX film *Into America's Wild*, narrated by Morgan Freeman; served on the President's Council for Sports, Fitness and Nutrition; and founded Blue Ridge Hiking Company, a Western North Carolina guiding service she began in 2008. Jennifer lives in Asheville, North Carolina, with her husband, Brew, and her children, Charlotte and Gus.